MEDICAL SCIENCE IN THE 21ST CENTURY

Sunset or New Dawn?

MEDICAL SCIENCE IN THE 21ST CENTURY

Sunset or New Dawn?

Desmond J Sheridan

Imperial College London, UK

Imperial College Press

ICP

Published by

Imperial College Press
57 Shelton Street
Covent Garden
London WC2H 9HE

Distributed by

World Scientific Publishing Co. Pte. Ltd.
5 Toh Tuck Link, Singapore 596224
USA office: 27 Warren Street, Suite 401-402, Hackensack, NJ 07601
UK office: 57 Shelton Street, Covent Garden, London WC2H 9HE

British Library Cataloguing-in-Publication Data
A catalogue record for this book is available from the British Library.

MEDICAL SCIENCE IN THE 21ST CENTURY
Sunset or New Dawn?

ISBN 978-1-84816-954-8

Typeset by Stallion Press
Email: enquiries@stallionpress.com

Printed in Singapore by Mainland Press Pte Ltd.

Contents

Preface

At the end of 2011, UK Prime Minister David Cameron met with a group of leading biomedical scientists and heads of pharmaceutical companies in Downing Street to discuss the future of the life sciences industry. This was clearly part of the government's response to a realisation that this industry is in trouble. Following a period of extraordinary successes during the 20th century in developing new drugs, which made it rich, big pharma now faces uncertainty with poor research performance and too few drugs under development. The government was stung earlier in the year by the closure of Pfizer's research centre in Sandwich and Astra's at Charnwood with the loss of thousands of highly paid jobs. The prime minister spoke about the government's recognition of the importance of the life sciences industry for the UK economy and of his government's commitment to retaining a strong foothold in the UK through tax incentives, easing regulation, making the health service more willing to take up new innovations and creating a number of technology and innovation centres. He also announced the intention to make patients' health service records available for research purposes.

It is a paradox of the early 21st century that an industry which enjoyed stunning success in the past should so quickly find itself in difficulty. However it would be a mistake to think that the industry is alone in its predicament. Medical science also enjoyed remarkable successes during the 20th century. Dramatic reductions in mortality caused by infectious diseases, heart disease and indeed conditions associated with most areas of medicine contributed to our current unprecedented longevity. However as the new century approached a decline began which continues today. Advances in biological science continue apace, but translating these into useful medical advances is widely acknowledged to be disappointing.

The social, political and economic factors in which this rise and fall of medical science occurred are complex and have resulted in unprecedented changes in the environment in which medical science operates. Health care costs have risen sharply in recent decades and much of this can be attributed to successes in treating illness. As a result, reforming the way care is delivered has become the new priority as efforts are made to find savings and increase efficiency and productivity. Clinical science, traditionally the generator of new ideas and priorities in biomedical science, has increasingly been seen as an expensive luxury in this new era and has been marginalised in efforts to find savings. As a result much of biomedical science is now far removed from the clinical coalface and far too little of it translates into patient benefits. It produces booming citation metrics to satisfy academic ratings, but has failed to generate the new avenues needed for therapeutic innovation.

Public attitudes towards medicine and science have also changed in recent decades. People are less deferential towards figures of authority and expect to be much more closely involved in decisions about their medical care. Patients' expectations and demands have also increased sharply as they have become better informed. At the same time well-publicised cases of medical mistakes and incompetence and fraudulent medical science have led some to question the reliability of medical ethics and professionalism and more generally their trust in science.

Thus, the 21st century finds medical science in decline, despite unprecedented advances in biological sciences. The emphasis of health economics in recent years has been to efficiently deliver that which is now possible. But this also tends to distract attention from the challenges we will face in the future and these are formidable. Globalisation makes the health of the world's population a matter of concern to us all. Air travel means that outbreaks of highly contagious infectious diseases on the far side of the planet can now threaten us within a matter of hours. Global health inequalities contribute to economic and political instability in countries far from our shores, but from which we are not immune. Rich countries face a demographic transition unique in human history as there are now more people over the age of 65 than under five. We already see the social, economic and political consequences of this as the retirement age increases in many countries. Meeting these challenges will require maintaining the efforts of medical science to find new ways to identify and prevent epidemics and much better treatments for chronic diseases that will reduce disability in later life.

In this book I explore the rise of medical science in the late 20th century, its history and how and why it was so successful. The decline which followed is now widely acknowledged, but it is important to try to understand the reasons for it: the radical changes to the environment in which it works, the stretched health budgets which have marginalised academic medicine in favour of a more efficient target driven service and the endless bureaucratic upheavals which stifle the curiosity and creativity which drive all science.

Is medical science destined for a final sunset? Or, as the Prime Minister's speech hinted, will the negative impact that the decline in medical science is having on the economy finally swing the pendulum in its favour? In a sense the question hangs in the balance for we appear truly ambivalent about medical science. On the one hand life sciences are hugely important for our economy; it is a powerful generator of foreign investment and economic productivity. On the other hand advances in medicine have contributed to rising health care costs and our recent efforts to control this by improving efficiency of delivery have served to undermine the medical component of life sciences on which its success depends. It is essential to reverse this negative and destructive attitude towards medical science, not just for the sake of the income generated by the life science industry, but also because improving health nationally and on a global scale is crucial for our future economic and political stability. We cannot expect millions of people to face longer working lives in the future unless we make it possible for them to do so by reducing the burden of chronic diseases and adult disability.

A new strategy to reverse the fortunes of life sciences has emerged in the last couple of years. This involves closer collaboration between industry and academia in an attempt to replicate the environment that was so successful in the 20th century. The keys to the success of this will be understanding how the complex creative process of medical science works and building the patient's bedside into the laboratory; not just as a place for basic scientists to visit occasionally or as a departmental label, but as the engine that drives the identification of the questions to ask of science. For this to happen, health care delivery will need to be revised to include the culture of scientific enquiry that underpinned past successes.

In writing this book I am conscious that many of the views I express may be met with disagreement or even outrage. However if it generates a greater awareness of the gradual insidious degradation of one of our most valuable social assets, and leads to thinking about the need to reverse this, it will have served a useful purpose.

1

The Rise and Fall of Medical Science in the 20ᵗʰ Century

The 20ᵗʰ century was a period of remarkable development in biomedical science. Advances made in this period were wide-ranging, surpassing anything achieved in earlier times in terms of scientific discoveries and their application in improving the treatment of diseases as well as the health of populations. The benefits derived during the 20ᵗʰ century affected all areas of health and were literally life-saving for millions of people worldwide. It would be all too easy to forget what life (and death) were like for so many before the introduction of antibiotics, for example, when 10% of pneumonia sufferers and almost all who contracted septicaemia, known then as 'blood poisoning', would have died. Deaths from cardio-vascular disease have been halved in most developed countries during the past quarter century, reflecting developments in treatment and prevention. Improved survival rates for cancer have proved more challenging, but even here substantial advances have been made and many cancers can now be cured. Indeed significant improvements have occurred in all fields of health care, contributing to the substantial increase in life expectancy we now enjoy. Despite this, anxieties about health are never far from the headlines. Well-publicised medical challenges, such as acquired hospital infections, antibiotic resistance and the poor experiences of some patients receiving treatment, understandably dominate the health agenda and obscure the extraordinary achievements of the past half century. Clearly the new challenges faced today will not be solved by taking comfort in

1

yesterday's successes. However if we lose sight of the underlying reasons for past medical successes we risk neglecting or discarding the foundations on which they were built and thereby the means of meeting our future needs. It is important therefore to understand the foundations of medical science, why medicine advanced so rapidly in the 20th century and why the rate of progress has been declining in recent years. What kinds of research led to these advances and what challenges have emerged to impede its progress?

The Foundations of Biomedical Science

Advances in science can always be traced back to developments in earlier times (Box 1.1) and the history of medicine is a very long one. There is a tradition among doctors of acknowledging and respecting the discoveries of their predecessors who made remarkable observations in recognising the symptoms and course of diseases. This reflects a genuine sense of indebtedness, particularly to the developments in medicine by the ancient Greeks which laid the foundations of Western medicine. It was these observations made by early Greek doctors, lost to Europe for many centuries but retained in the great Islamic libraries and later 'rediscovered' at the onset of the Enlightenment, which spearheaded the reawakening of modern medicine.

Healers practising before the modern era would have had a limited number of effective treatments available to them and many more that may have been more harmful than beneficial. We may be tempted to look on

Box 1.1

Foundations of Medical Science

- Value knowledge gained by predecessors
- Preserve knowledge for future generations
- Understand that knowledge transcends cultural boundaries
  — Discoveries are byproducts of knowledge
  — Discoveries are based on accumulated knowledge

these efforts with scepticism and even derision. Indeed when viewed through the retrospectoscope of our understanding today and our current needs, the therapeutic efforts of pre-modern physicians often appear worthless or worse. However this perspective can be misleading, especially as it fails to take account of the importance new observations and discoveries can have for future discoveries. For example, it is possible with current knowledge to judge that many of the treatments administered by pre-modern healers had little or no therapeutic value, but this does not invalidate or undervalue the contribution they made to science in recognising and understanding clinical signs and the courses of various diseases. In a modern context we would not judge everything that has been achieved in a particular area of medicine or by a group of scientists to be worthless if a treatment they hypothesised to be beneficial proved unsuccessful when tested in a clinical trial; we would still recognise that advances in understanding the disease process and new diagnostic techniques that led to its development could have great value. In other words, discoveries in medicine, as in science, have value quite separate from any products or treatments they lead to. Retaining and building on this knowledge through successive generations is a characteristic of scientifically progressive societies.

New Discoveries Depend on Accumulated Knowledge

Although the medical advances in the second half of the 20th century were quantitatively greater than in any previous period, they too were built on past achievements. In the case of developments in medical imaging, such as X-rays, ultrasound or magnetic resonance, all can be traced back through a succession of innovations to fundamental new discoveries in the 19th century. Advances in the treatment of heart disease in the second half of the 20th century were unprecedented, but here too the foundations were provided by earlier developments, such as the study of anatomy and William Harvey's discovery of blood circulation. The introduction of safe sewage disposal, which transformed public health in the 19th century, rested on an understanding of the nature of disease and the world of microbes and their effect on human health. Some historical writers have taken the view that medicine really only advanced in recent centuries with the discovery of bacteria, and that practice before that time was probably more harmful that beneficial.[1] Should we then discard the contributions of earlier doctors? There are several reasons why we should not. Firstly, because to do so would seem to accept a highly utilitarian view of medicine as seen through an economic lens focused on measurable performance that probably has its roots in the modern discipline of health economics. It sees benefit in terms of immediate health outcomes but ignores other less tangible contributions. Little is known about how effective or harmful most medical treatments were in the era before clinical trials and few would dispute that many were probably of little therapeutic value, and some even harmful. But it would be extremely simplistic to judge the practice of our predecessors in this way. In the modern world clinical trials allow us to accurately determine the ability of various treatments to relieve symptoms, prolong life or restore full health. But medicine has always been concerned with more than this. For example, hospice care for people who are dying is based primarily on providing comfort and relieving distress; continuing treatment aimed at curing a condition when there is little or no prospect of success would be a hindrance to that objective. In such circumstances, human contact and empathy, which recognise the dignity of the person, are the mainstays of support. The value of such care may be difficult to measure in economic terms but it has immense value in the broader human sense that would have been recognised as readily in ancient times as it is today. Thus, while early doctors had far fewer effective treatments than we enjoy today, they laid the foundations of a system of medicine which was crucial for the revival of European medicine during the Enlightenment after centuries of decline.

Early Healers Laid the Foundations for Modern Medicine

The history of healing probably extends back to the dawn of human consciousness and empathy. Evidence of practice, including the recognition of disease and bone setting, has been found in the Babylonian and Egyptian civilisations and medicine was also practised in ancient times in India and China. However it was developments of medicine in ancient Greece and the way it was documented that had the greatest impact on the development of Western medicine.[2] Doctors at the time were concerned not only with diagnosis and healing, but also with philosophy, ethics and the natural world. Achieving cures for their patients was clearly important and reinforced by severe penalties in the case of failure, as set out in Babylonian law around 1700 BC.[3] Diagnosis, and particularly the ability to predict the course of an illness, would also have had great value to politicians, military commanders and others holding positions of influence. Knowledge and understanding of disease through experience and example was therefore important and quite separate from drugs and other treatments. The Greeks developed dissection, initially limiting its practice to animals. However it was the spread of Greek culture to Alexandria where, under the rule of Ptolemy, sensitivities about the human body diminished, which allowed anatomical dissection to be extended to humans around 280 BC[2].

This is an early example of the process which would be crucial many centuries later in the revival of European medicine. These early doctors understood the importance of wide-ranging intellectual and practical skills, documentation and preservation of knowledge to ensure its transmission through generations and cultures so that we, their successors, could build on it to develop new knowledge through further study. Greek medicine continued to flourish during the Roman era, reaching its peak around the time of Galen (129–216 AD), whose works spread rapidly throughout the Roman world and remained widely influential for many centuries. With the collapse of the Roman Empire, the economies of Western Europe declined, and so too did medical practice. The Greek traditions were replaced by a return to spiritual healing and miracle cures. In contrast, the growth and spread of Islam in the south and east were accompanied by a rejuvenation of classical learning and this was initiated by the translation of Galenic and Greek texts into Arabic by several scholars, notably Hunain ibn Ishaq and his pupils. This transfer of knowledge stimulated a rapid expansion of medical writing in Arabic from the 10th to the 13th centuries. Perhaps the most important of these was Ibn Sina's *Canon of Medicine*, which was based on a deep understanding of Galen's work and shows a similar appreciation of philosophy and logic as well as medicine. It is still admired today for its clinical observation and teaching.[4,5]

Preservation of Knowledge through Successive Generations

The rise of medicine in Western Europe after the Dark Ages (500–1050 AD) was similarly based on the transfer of knowledge between cultures. Initially in southern Italy at Salerno, links with the Arab world influenced medical teaching. Constantine the African[6] began to translate Arabic texts into Latin from around 1060, leading to the reintroduction of Galenic learning. Similar knowledge transfer took place in Spain based on a major translation movement led by the Italian scholar, Gerard of Cremona[7] so that by about 1190 many of Galen's texts, as well as many Arabic medical texts had been translated. Gerard's translations also included works based on Aristotelian science as well as medical works. These introduced natural science into the medical curriculum in Europe and university medicine, which by 1400 was spreading throughout Western Europe.

European medicine began to change radically from the 17th century. Publication of Andreas Vesalius' *De Humani Corporis Fabrica* (On the Fabric of the Human Body) was a key moment in this. It represented a much more detailed approach to anatomical study based on greatly improved dissection methods and was widely published. More importantly, it was part of a scientific revolution that challenged the classical view of nature which included the concept that the body was composed of living essences that were self-determining. These new ideas proposed instead that all things were subject to the universal laws of nature and were supported by the discovery of the laws of physics as well as by the writings of philosophers such as René Descartes and Thomas Hobbes. This also led to a renewed interest in anatomy and the idea of the body as a machine, which was instrumental in advancing experimentation into how the body works and led directly to Harvey's discovery of blood circulation and the pump function of the heart. This mechanical view of nature initiated an astonishing expansion of anatomical and physiological research in the 18th and 19th centuries, which in turn led to the study of cell biology, molecular biology and genetics in the 20th century.

What does this tell us about the circumstances and conditions that lead to medical advances? Firstly, that recognition of the value of knowledge and the care taken to ensure its retention through generations has consistently provided later generations with the foundation on which rejuvenation and advances have occurred. The knowledge base during successful periods has been broad as well as grounded in clinical experience; in classical times it encompassed philosophy and ethics, in recent centuries natural sciences and most recently pure sciences. Secondly, when this culture is allowed to decline, as occurred after the fall of the Roman Empire and the collapse of classical education, it can take many generations for the knowledge base to recover. Thirdly, the ability to gather knowledge from other cultures and intellectual disciplines has been critical in reversing declines in the knowledge base, changing the direction of subsequent study and accelerating the speed of advances. What is striking about these three conditions is the fact that they all reflect the cultural characteristics of societies committed to education and learning (Box 1.2). They contain no specific elements of this or that curriculum, instead emphasising the importance of rigorous thinking across a wide range of subjects and an appetite to embrace new concepts and new disciplines. This commitment to the search for new knowledge, its documentation and preservation beyond the immediate needs of the day, has allowed medicine to advance not only in the 20th century, but throughout history. It would be a historic irony if we failed to maintain this commitment in the 21st century due to the short-term economic pressures we now face.

Box 1.2

Cultures Successful in Medical Science

- Medical science central to health protection
- Encouraging open enquiry
- Science based in, and led from, clinical experience
- Strong links to other sciences
- Training new medical scientists

The Search for New Knowledge and Understanding

Medical advances, like those in other areas of science, are based on taking what is known and building on it by adding new knowledge. This process of discovery is often referred to as 'research'. What is this process, and what do we mean by research? Research may mean a careful study to find known facts about some specific thing or person, but in science it usually has a more specific meaning; a systematic investigation of a subject to uncover new facts. In today's world, perhaps the most frequent form of research by individuals involves an internet search to find some piece of information, for example, the best replacement for a broken domestic appliance. However it is obvious that such a search is highly unlikely to reveal any new information about the type of appliance concerned or how to construct better machines. In that sense the research it is not original and does not seek to uncover new facts. In the public sphere 'market research' is probably what people encounter most frequently. This can be a valuable means of gathering information about aspects of human behaviour. For example, sales managers may wish to understand what attracts people to purchase a particular product in order to compete more effectively in the marketplace. But once again, it does not usually uncover any new information about human behaviour, the products involved or even about how competitive markets operate.

'Scientific research' might be considered a more suitable description of work that leads to new discoveries. But this term can also lead to misunderstandings. Firstly, research that seeks to discover new facts may involve areas that are not thought of as scientific, for example, research in areas such as history, archaeology or linguistics. Yet such work can be as significant and important in its contribution to society as anything in medicine or any other branch of science. Clearly, therefore, the term 'scientific' does not always distinguish research that is original from other forms of information gathering. Furthermore, many forms of research that might be described as 'scientific' may reveal nothing that is new. For example, statistical methods have greatly improved the accuracy of research, including market research, by ensuring that data is correctly sampled and of sufficient size to allow meaningful analysis. Likewise sophisticated biochemical analysis may be used to determine the quality and safety of products on sale to the public or to monitor air and water quality. All of these examples provide valuable information, but none may be intended or have any prospect of discovering any new facts. Similarly research into the way health care is delivered can, and has, led to valuable improvements in the efficiency with which care is provided, but does not lead to any new understanding of the nature of disease or to better diagnostic methods or treatments. Clearly, therefore, the term 'scientific' as currently used does not necessarily describe research that is either original or likely to lead to new discoveries.

The Focus of Medical Research has Changed

Does any of this matter? Should we be concerned about the way terminology is used and whether it changes? Some may say it matters little; it could be argued, for example, that all research has some value related to the reason for which it was carried out and that it is not the role of scientists to be concerned about the common use of language. Where it does matter however, is if such terminology affects our perception of the amount, character and quality of research being undertaken. This has special relevance for medical science, which has seen a marked change in the focus of its research resulting in a reduction in the effort devoted to seeking new treatments and understanding of disease in recent decades.

As I have said, advances in biomedical science during the 20th century have transformed medical care in many ways. Diagnostic methods are more sensitive and accurate; treatments are more effective and specific. They are also far more sophisticated as well as more widely available. These advances have also dramatically increased the demand for health care and the cost of its delivery. The task of regulating, managing and controlling these matters has become a major challenge for even the wealthiest of nations, who often struggle to contain costs while trying to achieve equity of availability for all. For this reason health care has become a major economic and political issue around the world. The French health insurance system delivers the best health care[8] according to the World Health Organisation (WHO), but it is over budget and faces cutbacks and reform. The British National Health Service (NHS) has been in a state of continuous reform since the 1980s, with further new radical reforms announced by the coalition government elected in 2010. The search for improvements in efficiency is put forward as a major driver for this despite the fact that the NHS was reported as the most efficient health system in the world by the Commonwealth Fund, an independent US foundation.[9] This contradiction has led some to suspect that political rather than economic motives are at work in the reform agenda.[10] Reform of the US health insurance system has also been one of the most contentious issues for several recent administrations.

Managing the economic and political tensions between expectations, availability and costs of health care therefore dramatically altered the focus of research in health care as the 21st century dawned. Market research to understand the expectations of patients and the public in general has become important for those tasked with managing health systems as well as for the politicians elected to oversee them. Measuring the performance of health workers as well as the units and systems in which they are organised is equally important. Research on health economics and policy has grown rapidly during the past 10–20 years, supported by several new specialist publications that have appeared in the same period. While this may provide useful information to direct and manage health care, it has little to do with discovering new diagnostic methods and treatments of disease. Furthermore, as delivery of health care becomes more complex, the need to measure various aspects of the process has increased, which in turn has shifted the focus of health workers away from the fundamental questions of how and why illnesses develop and how to treat them, to meeting and measuring delivery targets. Evidence of this shift in focus can be seen in many areas of clinical and academic medicine.

The Decline in Academic Medicine

The most striking evidence for a decline in academic medicine has been the sharp decline in recruitment of young clinical scientists in countries with a strong tradition of biomedical science. In the UK the recruitment of clinical lecturers fell by 52% between 2000 and 2006.[11] Some efforts to improve matters were made subsequently, but by 2009 the number in-post was still down by 43% compared to 2000. Similar changes have been reported in Europe[12,13] and the United States.[14] The decline in academic medicine is also evident in changes in the authorship of publications in medical journals. The contribution of clinical scientists to papers in life sciences research has fallen; by 2004, less than half of the workers in the fields of immunology, molecular biology or pharmacology had a medical degree, and most of those who did were over 55 years of age.[15] In addition, papers reporting original research are increasingly being replaced by articles dealing with health policy, health care delivery, quality of health care and derivative research based on previously published original work. Some issues of our medical journals that are ranked at the highest level in citation metrics often contain little or no original research,[16] which would have been rare 20 years ago. Furthermore, reports on global health written by or contributed to by health bodies such as the WHO often fail to register the contribution that medical science makes to improvements in health, or even its existence as a significant component of health care systems.[17] It is as if the economic pressures on health care have resulted in medical science paradoxically being perceived as an economic burden due to the increased costs associated with providing the new treatments and diagnostic methods it has achieved.[18] Consequently it now appears to be deliberately marginalised as a threat to health care in a new era of short-term economic imperatives.

It might seem surprising that medical science, which proved so successful in the recent past, should so quickly have fallen into decline. But perhaps it should not. The collapse of classical medicine lasted for many centuries before the Enlightenment brought about its revival, and it is only in recent times that medicine has enjoyed success or been considered a suitable occupation for a gentleman. Questions for the future will be whether medical science's present decline is a reflection of wider stresses in society and what these might be. Most sociologists and anthropologists who have studied the rise and fall of institutions and civilisations agree that how societies solve the problems they encounter is a key element in how they evolve. In the modern era science is the most important resource for this, and its effectiveness has come under close scrutiny in recent years. Recent economic studies have claimed that research productivity has been declining over the past three decades in most Western countries[19] and others point out that as societies develop and become more complex, solutions to the problems they encounter always involve increased cost, energy use and complexity.[20] This has led to the idea of decline based on the law of diminishing returns; as further investment becomes unaffordable, the institutions on which the society depended for survival degrade and decline follows.[20] Others point to political structures and rivalries to explain decline. In *Guns, Germs and Steel: The Fates of Human Societies*, Jared Diamond attributes the withdrawal from investing in ocean voyages and building sea-going ships in China during the 15th century to political rivalries and a highly centralised form of government.[21] But practical economics and defence strategy may also have played a part in that the predominant threats at the time came from land, as did most of China's trade. In *A Short History of Progress*, Ronald Wright describes failed civilisations as having fallen victim to 'progress traps', by which he means short-term successes that create new problems, which the society is then unwilling or unable to resolve. He sees many of the great monuments of extinct civilisations in our deserts and jungles today as evidence of past progress traps and he likens them to the black boxes of crashed airliners.[22] But perhaps a more striking analogy from our time might be the re-emergence of gross inequalities in wealth in some countries in recent years.

Are any of these mechanisms behind the decline in medical science? Economic pressures on health care budgets are certainly cited as a major problem, and economists point to diminishing returns on research investment. But these are often presented in economic models as undifferentiated blocks of information and can be misleading. For example, health budgets are indeed stretched, but medical science has achieved improvements in health and longevity during the past century never before experienced by humanity and, with the exception of the United States, this has occurred with modest increases in expenditure when expressed in terms of gross domestic product (GDP). More often than not, arguments about health budgets are really about how societies should pay for health care, how it can be most efficiently delivered and whether it should be provided on a community basis or by individuals. In regard to research productivity, information tends to be presented as if all forms of research were the same. But what is often classified as research in this context has nothing to do with scientific discovery. For example, neither market research nor routine work carried out during the development of products to meet regulatory requirements are undertaken to seek new scientific knowledge, but both add huge costs to what economists refer to as 'research budgets'. In contrast, many valuable advances have been made in low-cost laboratories by scientists driven by curiosity. Some of these scientists have been criticised for failing to capture the commercial value of their work. On the other hand, it is often the accumulation of business and competitive bureaucracies that overload research budgets and degrade efficiency.

This matters for medical science because many of its most important contributions have been made by clinical scientists working across the disciplines of medical practice and laboratory science, often in low-cost settings. Examples include the early work on the development of artificial joints[23] and coronary care units.[24] These small beginnings led to major worldwide advances in the treatment of osteoarthritis and acute coronary syndromes. The early work met with official objections and poor support, and was only possible due to the motivation of the key clinical scientists and a degree of budgetary flexibility that has long since disappeared. It is the loss of this element of biomedical research — namely the engagement of our brightest clinicians, energised by the suffering of patients and the limitations of medicine to help them, in finding better ways to diagnose and treat diseases — that I believe is at the root of its decline.

Thus, research in health care continues apace, but its character has changed dramatically during the past 20 years to reflect the new economic and political environment of health care delivery. We have major investments in biological laboratories that are effectively disconnected from the clinical arena on the one hand and on the other pragmatic research related to cost effectiveness and efficiency. Both undoubtedly have uses, but they struggle to produce any new therapies or diagnostic methods. This lack of innovation poses the most serious risk facing medical science in the 21st century. As we have seen, recognising the value of scientific knowledge and building on it to make new discoveries has been fundamental to advancing medical science. This requires an infrastructure in which medical practice can be combined with original scientific enquiry related to clinical experience. The risks for biomedical science are that the benefits it has produced are obscured by our present economic and political challenges and that its infrastructure has come to be viewed as costly and unaffordable in an era when short-term economics drives the health care agenda. It is all the more important therefore to consider what we mean by research and what research is being undertaken. We must also recognise that however much we invest in research, it is only through original scientific enquiry into diseases and their treatment that medical advances can be made.

Summary and Conclusions

Medical science made unprecedented advances during the 20th century that contributed to the substantial improvements in health and life expectancy we now enjoy. The origins of this success can be traced back to the foundations of medical science laid in the classical Greek period. Much of that work was translated into Arabic and was preserved in Islamic culture during the Dark Ages in Europe, 500–1050 AD. Later translated into Latin from Arabic, this knowledge was critical for the revival of medicine during the Enlightenment. The scientific revolution during the 17th century paved the way for a more objective and rational approach to science which sparked a dramatic expansion of anatomical and physiological research in the 18th and 19th centuries, and molecular biology and genetics during the 20th century. Preserving knowledge and building on it through new discoveries by successive generations were fundamental to this scientific progress.

These successes led to advances in diagnostic methods and therapies and to dramatic improvements in health and longevity. They also contributed to increased health costs, leading some to consider medical science as a burden on health care which needed to be controlled. As a result, the focus of research began to shift from about 1980 away from medical science in favour of measurements of the quality of care and efficiency. Recruitment of young clinical scientists has fallen sharply and research into the context of clinical practice has declined.

Reactions to these circumstances has varied; some regard what they see as the 'publish or perish' culture of the past as wasteful, while others openly view innovation as a threat to efficient health care delivery.[18] Some have thought the problem of recruiting young scientists to be one of logistics and bureaucracy,[25] however the extent and speed of the decline indicates a more fundamental change. It is as if confidence in medical science to find solutions to health problems has waned and we now look elsewhere for answers.

It is a historic irony that the rapid ascent of medical science in the 20th century should be matched by the speed of its decline in the 21st. There are signs that the risks this poses to our health and prosperity are being recognised and alarm bells are being rung.[26] As yet it is unclear as to whether they will be heard. What is clear is that medical science faces a critical period during the 21st century which is likely to be as interesting and important as any time in its history.

References

1. Wootton, D., *Bad Medicine: Doctors Doing Harm Since Hippocrites*. Oxford University Press, Oxford, 2006.
2. Nutton, V., The rise of medicine, in *The Cambridge Illustrated History of Medicine*, Ed. by Porter, R., Cambridge University Press, Cambridge, 1996. p. 52–81.
3. Spiegel, A.D. and Springer, C.R., Babylonian medicine, managed care and Codex Hammurabi, circa 1700 B.C. *J. Community Health*, 1997; 22(1), 69–89.
4. Shoja, M.M., Tubbs, R.S., Loukas, M., *et al.*, Vasovagal syncope in the Canon of Avicenna: the first mention of carotid artery hypersensitivity. *Int. J. Cardiol.*, 2009; 134(3), 297–301.
5. Aciduman, A., Arda, B., Ozaktürk, F.G., *et al.*, What does Al-Qanun Fi Al-Tibb (the Canon of Medicine) say on head injuries? *Neurosurg. Rev.*, 2009; 32(3), 255–263.
6. Constantine the African. Science Museum website. http://www.sciencemuseum. org.uk/broughttolife/people/constantinetheafrican.aspx. Accessed 5 July 2012.
7. Gerard of Cremona. Science Museum website. http://www.sciencemuseum. org.uk/broughttolife/people/gerardofcremona.aspx. Accessed 5 July 2012.
8. WHO, World health report 2000. Health systems: improving performance. WHO, Geneva, 2001. www.who.int/whr/2000/en/index.html. Accessed 5 July 2012.
9. Tanne, J.H., US comes last in international comparison of health systems. *BMJ*, 2007; 334, 1078.
10. Pickstone, J., The rule of ignorance: a polemic on medicine, English health service policy, and history. *BMJ*, 2011; 342, 633–634.
11. Fitzpatrick, S., for the Medical Schools Council. A survey of staffing levels of medical clinical academics in UK medical schools as at 31 July 2009.

http://www.medschools.ac.uk/AboutUs/Projects/Documents/Clinical%20 Academic%20Staff%20Survey%202010.pdf. Accessed 4 July 2012.

12. Van Der Meer, J.W., The detection and cultivation of the scientific talent of young doctors. *Verh. K. Acad. Geneeskd. Belg.*, 2005; 67, 67–72.

13. Ludvigsson, J.F., Hard times for Swedish physicians-researchers. *Nature,* 2005; 434, 542.

14. Ley, T.J. and Rosenberg, L.E., The physician-scientist career pipeline in 2005: build it, and they will come. *JAMA*, 2005; 294, 1343–1351.

15. Ioannidis, J.P.A., Academic medicine: the evidence base. *BMJ*, 2004; 329, 789–791.

16. See, for example, *BMJ*, 26 March 2011; 342.

17. European Observatory on Health Systems and Policies, Health systems in transition. http://www.euro.who.int/en/home/projects/observatory/publications/health-system-profiles-hits/full-list-of-hits. Accessed 4 July 2012.

18. Gabbay, J. and Walley, T., Introducing new health interventions. *BMJ*, 2006; 332, 64–65.

19. Everson, R., Patents, R&D and invention potential: international evidence. *Amer. Econ. Rev.*, 1993; 83, 463–468.

20. Tainter, J.A., Complexity, problem solving, and sustainable societies, in *Complexity, Problem Solving, and Sustainable Societies*, Ed. by Costanza, R., Segura, O. and Martinez-Alier, J., Island Press, Washington D.C., 1996.

21. Diamond, J.A., *Guns, Germs, and Steel: The Fates of Human Societies*. W.W. Norton & Co., New York, 1997.

22. Wright, R., *A Short History of Progress*. Avalon Publishing Group, New York, 2004.

23. McKee, G.K., The Norwich method of total hip replacement: development and main indications, *Ann. R. Coll. Surg. Engl.*, 1974; 54(2), 53–62.

24. Julian, D.G., The evolution of the coronary care unit. *Cardiovasc. Res.*, 2001; 51, 621–624.

25. Modernising Medical Careers, Medically- and dentally-qualified academic staff: recommendations for training the researchers and educators of the future. Report of the Academic Careers Sub-committee of Modernising Medical Careers and the UK Clinical Research Collaboration, March 2005. http://www.ukcrc.org/index.aspx?0=3146. Accessed 5 July 2012.

26. Academy of Medical Sciences, Clinical academic medicine in jeopardy: recommendations for change. June 2002. http://www.acmedsci.ac.uk/p99puid25.html. Accessed 5 July 2012.

2

Advances in Medicine: How Are They Made?

When a leading journal recently called for papers in my area of interest I should have been pleased, but instead I felt a certain disappointment. When a generous funder of medical research announced a major new investment in cell regeneration, my pleasure was also tinged with a feeling of concern about whether this is the way to do science. Indeed both of my reactions arise from a sense that neither approach reflects an understanding of the way science actually works. I have no doubt that both endeavours will have some positive results in one way or another, and that many would regard my reaction as lacking in generosity. To explain why my response was less than fulsome, I should clarify that the call for papers was restricted to papers that focus on clinical trials that are likely to have a significant impact on clinical practice. While this appears to be an entirely appropriate way to publish work that will interest health workers and promote good clinical practice, I immediately thought of all the momentous scientific discoveries that would be excluded by such a qualifier. How would the editor know whether a piece of work would influence clinical practice when very often scientists themselves may not be able to foresee what influence their work might have? Did the editor think that only clinical trials could influence clinical practice? Regarding the generous offer of grant support, I sensed a wish to manage research efficiently and in a direction the funder felt was necessary to be successful. Prioritising efficiency and areas of need both seem entirely rational and sensible ways to better manage and direct science. However I could not help doubting whether the process of scientific discovery is capable of responding to such efforts, however well intentioned. This raises the question, how are scientific discoveries made? What processes are involved in gathering new knowledge that leads to them? Medical science has achieved great successes in the 20th century, but now appears to be in decline. What initiated these successes at the level of the working scientist and what processes led to their introduction into clinical practice? What can this teach us about the appropriate value to place on discoveries and how best to encourage and support further breakthroughs?

What Works in Biomedical Science?

To answer these questions it is helpful to consider how some of the diagnostic techniques and treatments that are widely used in medicine today were developed. The electrocardiogram (ECG) is a routine workhorse found in every hospital and in almost all GP practices. It provides information about the electrical properties of the heart as each beat is generated. From this, clinicians can ascertain the health of the heart and the stability of its rhythm, two attributes that are helpful in diagnosing a wide range of conditions, including the likelihood of heart attacks. The impact of the ECG on medicine has been immense and today practice without it would be hard to envisage. The data from ECGs has also been valuable in epidemiological studies to determine the prevalence of heart disease and to study the effect of preventive measures. Indeed the ECG has contributed significantly to the reduction in deaths from coronary disease achieved over the past decades. And yet, when the technique for capturing ECG data was pioneered in humans by Augustus Waller in 1887[1] he noted that he did not think it would play much role in hospital practice.

Advances in Diagnostic Methods: Triggers and Cycles

Although Waller's method was relatively imprecise, Willem Einthoven, who saw him demonstrate it, quickly implemented a more sensitive recording method using the string galvanometer. This greatly improved the quality of ECG data and as a result electrocardiography became much more widely available to physiologists and clinicians. For generations, countless contributions were made to medical science through interpreting ECG data from both normal subjects and patients with various forms of heart disease (Figure 2.1). This led to greatly improved methods for diagnosing arrhythmias, coronary heart disease, heart block and indeed almost all forms of heart disease. In science, new discoveries always lead to new questions, and so too in medicine each new understanding of a disease or its diagnosis always leads to new therapeutic challenges. For example, the ability to diagnose arrhythmias accurately led to an improved understanding of their underlying causes, and from that to the need for portable monitoring systems and to therapies such as anti-arrhythmic drugs and the cardiac defibrillator. The ECG was also the key to accurately diagnosing heart block, which in turn led to the development of pacemakers. Perhaps most importantly, the ECG allowed much more accurate diagnosis of myocardial infarction (heart attack) and this was essential for research that identified the causes of heart attacks, based on accurate clinical diagnosis and careful pathological study. This in turn was critical for the host of treatments and preventions that led to such a dramatic reduction in heart attacks and deaths later in the 20th century.

The above example illustrates how an initial discovery can become such a major contributor to advances in medicine through successive and continuous development (Figure 2.1). A significant feature of many scientific advances is the fact that the future potential of their initial discovery was not foreseen by anyone involved in it. Its importance and value could not therefore be measured in any meaningful way. A second significant feature is that subsequent developments were dependent on findings obtained from the initial discovery, and so they too could not have been predicted. These characteristics, far from being unusual, are in fact typical of most discoveries.

The ability to image the internal organs of patients was a major advance of the 20th century. The use of ultrasound had its origin in the discovery of piezoelectricity by the Curie brothers, Pierre and Jacques, in 1880 (Figure 2.2). The Curies' initial experiments were designed to show that compression of crystal structures would generate a voltage across them. They later tested the reverse hypothesis, that the application of a

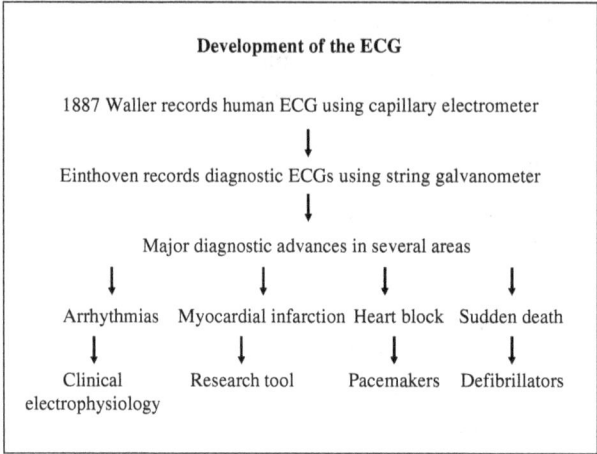

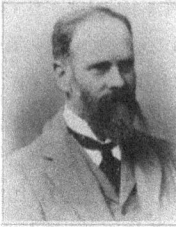

Figure 2.1.   The first recording of the electrocardiogram in a human by Augustus Waller was reported in 1887. Although initially not considered, even by Waller, likely to be of much use in clinical practice, it seeded a revolution in diagnostic and therapeutic developments by subsequent generations of scientists and clinicians. Each advance depended on earlier discoveries and was usually motivated by them. This pattern illustrates the incremental and contingent nature of advances and highlights the difficulty of making discoveries in science and measuring their value. It also illustrates the often inherent unpredictability of scientific advances.

voltage to crystals would alter their shape,[2] which is the basis for producing ultrasound. Initially used in industry to examine the internal structure of materials, two Swedish clinical scientists, Inge Edler and Carl Hellmuth Hertz, demonstrated the potential use of ultrasound in humans using a borrowed industrial machine. This was the stimulus which led to advances in transducer technology and the application of computer techniques to develop modern systems. Similarly, the discovery of X-rays by Wilhelm Roentgen in 1895 was serendipitous (Figure 2.3). He observed that a screen covered in fluorescent material was illuminated during experiments in which the source of rays he was working on was covered and the room was darkened, an effect that was purely accidental. From this he was able to deduce that the rays must have been able to penetrate several barriers to reach the screen. Later experiments confirmed that a number of objects could be penetrated by these rays.[3] The first post-mortem X-rays, including angiograms (images of the heart and circulation), soon followed and soon after came a rapid expansion in diagnostic radiology in the early

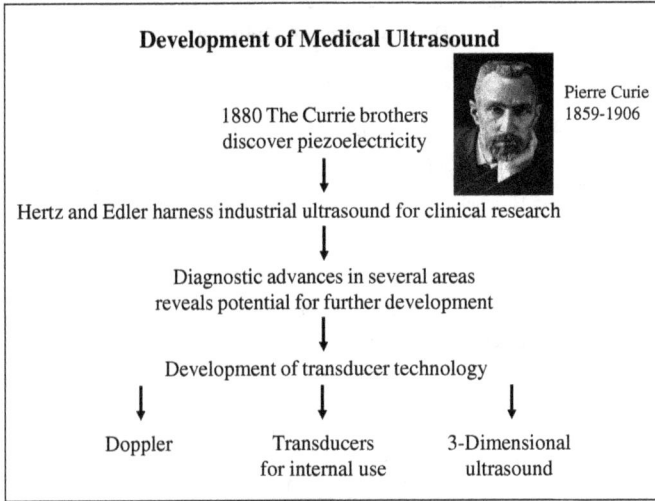

Development of Medical Ultrasound

1880 The Currie brothers
discover piezoelectricity

Pierre Curie
1859-1906

↓

Hertz and Edler harness industrial ultrasound for clinical research

↓

Diagnostic advances in several areas
reveals potential for further development

↓

Development of transducer technology

↓   ↓   ↓

Doppler   Transducers   3-Dimensional
for internal use   ultrasound

Figure 2.2. Developments in medical imaging depended on discoveries in physics in the 19th century. Ultrasound was based on the discovery of piezoelectricity by the Curie brothers in 1880. Two clinical scientists envisaged its possible use for imaging patients and demonstrated its potential using a borrowed industrial machine. This quickly led to development of specialised transducers for a range of clinical uses. Application of wave analysis allowed blood flow velocity to be measured and signal processing to the introduction of three dimensional ultrasound.

part of the 20th century. It is hard to think of any area of medicine that has not been greatly advanced by radiology. It was crucial for the introduction of angiography, which in turn led to vascular surgery, including coronary bypass operations, as well as angioplasty and coronary stenting.

Progress is Incremental and Contingent

These examples illustrate the sequential nature of discovery. It was more than half a century after the discovery of ultrasound before its potential for medical imaging was considered. Although Roentgen quickly understood the potential of X-rays for medical use, even here the extent to which radiology would transform medicine could not have been foreseen. The above examples also show how difficult, indeed impossible, it is to appreciate the value of new discoveries when they are first made. Both of these developments also depended on collaboration between clinicians and scientists in other fields, in this case physics. Further, these

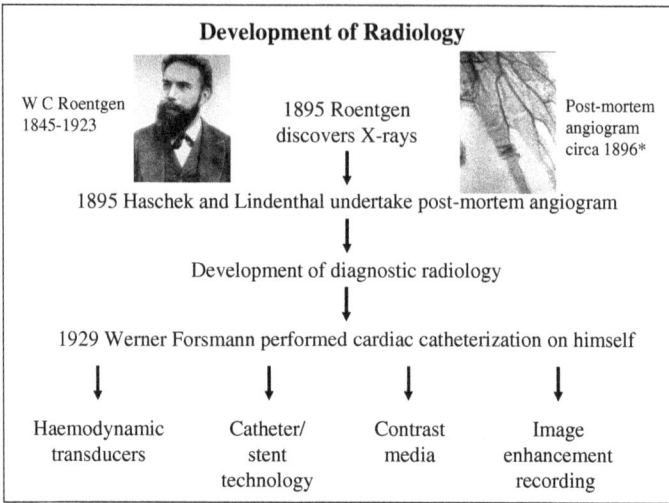

Figure 2.3.   Roentgen's serendipitous discovery of X-rays in 1895 was rapidly followed by tests of its possible use to image internal body structures, not only of bone but also of blood vessels as illustrated by the first post mortem angiogram in 1895. The diagnostic value of X-rays was established in the 20th century based on clinical experience in practice as its use spread worldwide. Angiography (imaging the heart blood vessels) permitted the diagnosis of coronary artery disease. This in turn led to bypass surgery and later angioplasty and stenting. (*From *Wien.Klin.Wochenschr.*1896, 9:63, with permission.)

examples also show how many discoveries of great importance are accidental and unplanned. The key to success is the ability of the scientist who made the initial observation to capture its significance and to investigate it further, for which training in the detection and analysis of new phenomena is essential. The successful scientist must also have a strong innate curiosity and the resources of time and materials for further study. Scientists familiar with the process of discovery have long been aware of the importance of these characteristics, as exemplified by the words of Louis Pasteur in his lecture at the University of Lille in 1854, 'in the fields of observation, chance favours only the prepared mind'. However this now runs counter to modern trends for managed efficiency and directed work and is increasingly difficult to accommodate in many organisations.[4] The discoveries of both ultrasound and X-rays also show the importance of knowledge transfer between medicine and other sciences which, as I discussed in Chapter 1, has been a feature of medical advances throughout history.

Discovery of New Drugs and Rediscovery of Old Drugs

Innovation in drug development can also be seen as relying on previous discoveries. The development of β-blockers was based on a new understanding of the autonomic nervous system and receptor pharmacology. The discovery of β-adrenoreceptors soon led to a search for targets to block them, and thence to early β-blockers such as propranolol. Subsequently the identification of β-receptor subtypes led to the development of more specific β-blockers with improved efficacy. But perhaps the most interesting aspect of β-blocker development relates to the observation that chronic overstimulation of the adrenergic system is an important feature of congestive cardiac failure and has an adverse effect on its prognosis. This discovery was made several years after the introduction of β-blockers and led to clinical trials that demonstrated the ability of β-blockers to improve survival in patients with heart failure, which in turn led to their introduction into treatment. These discoveries were made many years after the introduction of β-blockers, which at that time were contraindicated for use in patients with heart failure. It is interesting to reflect that while β-blockers are now being superseded by more effective drugs for the treatment of hypertension, they may in time come to be used most frequently to treat a condition for which they were contraindicated at the time they were introduced. This again underlines the continuous, incremental and unpredictable course that advances take and how this makes the task of accurately valuing them at the point of discovery difficult. It also shows how discoveries in one area of medical science can lead to advances in other disciplines.

One of the 20th century's most important and interesting advances was the 'rediscovery' of aspirin for the treatment of circulatory diseases. Willow bark has been used since ancient times and salicin was extracted from it in 1829. Aspirin was later synthesised and introduced as an empirical analgesic, and so it remained for almost a century. Clarification that almost all heart attacks are caused by coronary thrombosis was achieved in the 1970s and the ability of aspirin to inhibit platelets, a key element of the thrombotic process, was discovered in 1971.[5] These discoveries led to the hypothesis that aspirin might be useful in preventing heart attacks, which was later confirmed in large clinical trials.[6] This example shows how new knowledge can have a wide-ranging impact and how a better understanding of diseases and how medicines work can transform the value of already available drugs. It also illustrates that advances can be made from discoveries of all kinds; well-designed clinical trials can be just as important as laboratory-based science. We again see that the process of discovery is incremental and depends on the ongoing generation of new knowledge, which makes it difficult to direct the process in any meaningful way.

Advances in Clinical Practice: Bench to Bedside and Bedside to Bench

These processes of discovery also apply to clinical practice. The history of coronary care units (CCUs) illustrates this well and is worth describing in some detail (Figure 2.4). CCUs were introduced in the 1960s to manage heart attack patients.[7] In the years that followed there was much discussion about the value of CCUs and many argued that they were not cost effective based on studies of survival and their running costs.[8,9] No attempt was made in these studies to measure the contribution these units made to the growth of knowledge and improvements in the treatment of coronary disease that followed. However, the history of advances in the treatment of coronary heart disease that followed the introduction of CCUs clearly shows the limitations of that approach. These units proved extraordinarily effective in unravelling the natural history and cause of heart attacks and their complications.

As recently as 1972 there was controversy about whether coronary thrombosis was the cause of heart attacks or a consequence of them.[10,11] Collecting clinical histories from patients treated at home and in hospital and correlating these with their progress while being carefully monitored in CCUs permitted a detailed understanding of events from the onset of heart attacks. This was crucial to understanding the link between chest pain and sudden cardiac death and the need for urgent medical attention.[12] CCUs were particularly important in later clarifying the distinction between heart attacks, unstable angina and acute coronary syndromes, which led to the understanding that myocardial infarction could be prevented or mitigated by prompt treatment. The introduction of coronary angiography to clarify the diagnosis in patients also resolved and explained the controversy about coronary thrombosis. It confirmed that almost all patients with heart attacks had coronary thrombosis when

Coronary Care Units

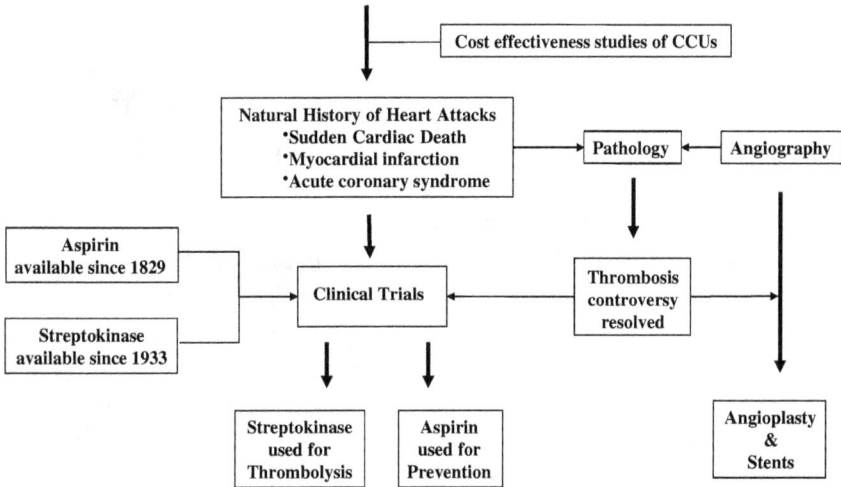

Figure 2.4. Coronary care units were introduced in the 1960s to care for patients suffering heart attacks. The intensive monitoring of patients by specially trained staff provided an ideal opportunity for the study of coronary disease and this contributed to the rapid development in understanding its clinical course, pathology and underlying causes. This in turn was instrumental in advancing treatment and prevention. The intensive monitoring on CCUs required greater investment than for routine ward care or treatment at home. This prompted concerns about their cost effectiveness and studies to assess this were carried out, some comparing their cost effectiveness with prevention programs. These studies were performed at a time when the scientific contributions of CCUs could not have been foreseen and so none attempted to include any value related to them. Failure to consider scientific contributions is a common failing in health economic assessments of clinical programs and risks damaging academic medicine.

examined within an hour of onset, but this fell rapidly to about 50% when examined 12–24 hours later,[13,14] indicating that in many patients spontaneous breakdown of the thrombus occurs, although usually too late to protect their hearts. This understanding of the pathology of coronary heart disease was crucial for the introduction of thrombolysis (a clot-busting treatment) and aspirin. CCUs brought together the perfect environment to facilitate a wider study of heart attacks and it is inconceivable that the rapid progress achieved would have been possible without them. They also, for the first time, allowed close monitoring of patients' heart rhythms, which helped to identify ventricular fibrillation as a frequent and reversible cause of sudden cardiac death, often within minutes of the onset of symptoms. In other words, CCUs made great contributions to the rapid advances in treating coronary heart disease during the second half of the 20th century. It would be difficult now to measure the value of this contribution, and to my knowledge this has not been attempted. How much more difficult would it have been to accurately ascertain the eventual value of CCUs so soon after their introduction at a time when none of these benefits could have been foreseen? The health economic studies available at the time made no attempt to assign any value to the information CCUs could contribute;[8,9] some compared the cost/benefit of CCUs in prevention versus other treatment strategies[9] without appearing to realise the interdependence between better knowledge and better prevention strategies. In other words, prevention strategies would never have been possible without the advances made in understanding the natural history and pathology of coronary heart disease, to which the CCU was a major contributor.

These examples illustrate several important features of the discovery process which have important implications for preserving and sustaining it. It is clear that many discoveries are made unexpectedly. This is especially important to appreciate at a time when we have seen dramatic changes in the way in which work is organised in the developed world. The 20th century has seen the widespread introduction of management systems to improve the efficiency of organisations. Assembly lines and modern call centres are examples that have greatly improved the efficiency of repetitive work. The basis for these is that by providing a defined and limited number of work steps to be followed, operatives become practiced and more efficient. These systems are also designed to replace the intellectual input of operators with rules and guidelines. This approach has undoubtedly increased the productivity of many of our industries.

More recently assembly line methods have also been successfully introduced in some areas of science. Perhaps the best and most widely known example is the mapping of the three billion base pairs that make up the human genome. This information will be invaluable in the decades ahead as a resource for scientists around the world in supporting a wide range of genetic studies. Identifying the sequence of three billion amino acids was a huge task undertaken by several laboratories in a global collaboration. It required careful coordination, quality control and data management across several groups of workers to achieve its goal. It was however largely a technological and organisational success rather than a scientific one in that the work was intended to document the details of what was already known and understood rather than make new discoveries. The undertaking was akin to building a new global library to support biological sciences and, although of great value as such, it would be wrong to view its construction as an example of the way original science needs to be conducted.

Workers undertaking repetitive tasks, however sophisticated the technology used, are not ideally placed to undertake original scientific enquiry. And yet this approach to science is being increasingly adopted, particularly in the pharmaceutical industry, where large numbers of science graduates are engaged in repetitive screening tasks in the search for new drugs or in testing for adverse effects to satisfy ever-increasing regulatory requirements. This is undoubtedly important work, but it should not be confused with original scientific enquiry. In all of the sciences, key discoveries on which future advances depend are often unplanned, arising accidentally and unexpectedly. Capturing these discoveries requires that the observer is trained in analysing original phenomena and has the opportunity to do so. This requires a particular form of training in which the capacity for original and critical thinking is developed. It also acknowledges that such work must be organised in a manner that allows the scientist to prioritise and lead the direction of travel, with sufficient leeway to permit new avenues to be explored when necessary.

Advances frequently occur as a result of cycles of multiple steps in discovery, each dependent on new knowledge arising in an earlier cycle. Descriptions of the way this occurs tend to oversimplify the route followed, as if it were pre-planned. But this can be misleading as it often reflects an attempt by the scientist involved to present a coherent description of the work when writing about it later. In practice, the future course of work cannot be decided well in advance as it needs to evolve in light of new experimental results. Flexibility of thought and of future planning is a fundamental requirement to allow original scientific research to flourish. This might well appear inefficient in some management systems and, if the need for such an approach is not properly understood, risks being stifled by inappropriate and over-zealous efforts to achieve greater efficiency.

The course that advances take is often unpredictable and in the early stages their importance and value may not be fully apparent. The increasing cost of health care has led to increased interest in the cost/benefit assessment of new treatments, often referred to as health technology assessment (HTA). While comparison of the costs and benefits of established therapies is relatively uncomplicated, measuring the value of new treatments or diagnostic methods can be extremely complicated. Some may have the potential to accelerate progress in the management of a disease in ways not apparent in the early stages of their development. Economic assessments are increasingly influential in guiding health policy. However HTAs risk damaging medical science if carried out prematurely and inappropriately when the full value of medical research cannot be properly assessed. This was demonstrated clearly in several early studies of the cost effectiveness of CCUs.

Advances in one area of science can dramatically impact other areas and the facility for interdisciplinary research is important for rapid cross-fertilisation. Since ancient times this has been a significant factor in scientific and medical advances. In the modern era such advances require that clinical scientists are able to collaborate with scientists in other disciplines. The examples given in this chapter show that this collaboration needs to operate in both directions; unidirectional models of biomedical science, in which clinicians are tasked with taking forward into practice discoveries made in other areas of science, would have inhibited such collaboration. Some clinicians involved in practice and familiar with its challenges need to be involved in basic science in order to give it direction and to capture potential advances in a timely manner. The idea that clinicians should be restricted to undertaking 'research involving patients' is far too simplistic and runs counter to all experience.

New advances in medicine can be initiated by discoveries in any specialism or area of expertise; careful clinical observation, well-designed clinical trials, new technical diagnostic methods or the most up to date genetic analysis can all be triggers for a spurt of knowledge growth. The 'rediscovery' of aspirin for treating coronary heart disease depended on understanding the role of thrombosis in causing heart attacks. This in turn required accurate diagnosis in conjunction with careful pathological studies. Indeed understanding the natural history and causes of disease is a prerequisite for all therapeutic advances. Close monitoring of patients on coronary care units was intended to improve treatment; but it also resulted in a much better understanding of acute coronary syndromes, which was the key stimulus for many advances in treatment that would follow. This underlines the important role clinicians have, not just as passive recipients of discoveries made in the laboratory, but of guiding basic research to address important clinical challenges.

Thus many, if not most, scientific discoveries are made unexpectedly rather than by successfully reaching predefined end points. This makes discovery a difficult process to manage or direct. In addition, many discoveries are made in what might be described as commercially naive conditions, where there is no prior sense of their likely financial value and their commercial worth may not be appreciated for some time. This can have both positive and negative effects. On the negative side, the researchers and institutions involved in a discovery may miss out on the financial benefits to be gained from patent rights and licencing agreements. Taxpayers who have funded the research may also miss out if the commercial exploitation moves abroad and the resulting profits and taxes follow. There is no doubt that this has been a sensitive issue in some countries and has led to the introduction of greater commercial awareness among academic institutions and health care providers. On the positive side, societies and, in the case of medical science, patients benefit from new discoveries irrespective of where the profits are reaped. Furthermore, research that is undertaken primarily to generate profits is also burdened with a large commercial bureaucracy, such as maintaining secrecy to protect information property and managing research so that it fits with the business strategy of the company, rather than simply seeking to generate new knowledge. This need to meet targets set by specific business considerations often obviates the possibility of pursuing alternate lines of enquiry which might otherwise be fruitful. A large commercial bureaucracy also adds labour and running costs to the research, while in all likelihood reducing the prospects of new discoveries.

Thus, open scientific research, in which the direction of enquiry is driven by science itself and influenced by emerging new knowledge rather than by commercial or other objectives, is more in keeping with the way new discoveries are made. I suggest that it is also likely to be more cost effective when its productivity is assessed in terms of new knowledge that leads to benefits to society when measured over time. I am not aware of any studies that have compared the productivity of open, unrestricted research with commercially-directed research. Any such study would need to be based on a long-term view in order to capture the downstream value that new knowledge has on the research and discoveries that it contributes to. This is an important question for biomedical science today. The decline in advances in medical science over the past few decades has been accompanied by marked increases in the commercial influences surrounding it and by closer management and direction to meet predefined strategic business objectives. Is it possible that we are stifling the original creativity of our budding young scientists by demands to meet managerial rather than scientific objectives?

Summary and Conclusions

Advances in medical science result from complex sequences of discovery. These sequences are incremental and contingent on surges of progress often triggered by key observations. They require scientists, clinical and non-clinical, who are trained in detecting and analysing new phenomena and who have the resources and flexibility to pursue them. The potential uses of discoveries are often unclear at the time they are made and attempts to apply premature cost/benefit studies to them are likely to be misleading and destructive.

Efforts to manage and direct health care have intensified in recent years in the pursuit of increased clinical efficiency. This has diverted clinicians away from original scientific research in favour of higher clinical through-put. The editors' call for papers and the grant funder's announcement discussed at the beginning of this chapter seem to me to reflect a similar attempt to better manage and direct science. However well intentioned they may be in seeking to promote more rapid clinical advances, they misunderstand the manner in which science works and risk exacerbating the already weakened state of biomedical science.

Original science does not operate as a simple rules-based system and attempts to manage it in such a manner risk extinguishing the element of creativity on which it depends. Restoring medical science to its former position of strength requires physician scientists who are able to work in a culture that understands and encourages the search for new knowledge and provides the flexibility for them to pursue their enquiries. Both are needed; trained physician scientists and a clinical base that welcomes and supports a culture of scientific enquiry.

References

1. Waller, A.D., A demonstration on man of electromotive changes that accompany the heart's beat. *J. Physiol.*, 1887; 8, 229–234.
2. Duck, F., The electrical expansion of quartz by Jacques and Pierre Curie. *Ultrasound*, 2009; 17, 197.
3. Roentgen's discovery of the X-ray. British Library website. http://www.bl.uk/learning/artimages/bodies/xray/roentgen.html. Accessed 5 July 2012.
4. Streskopf, M.K., Observation and cognition: how serendipity provides the building blocks for scientific discovery. *ILAR Journal*, 2005; 46, 332–337.
5. Ferreira, S.H., Moncada, S. and Vane, J.R., Indomethicin and aspirin abolish prostaglandin release from the spleen. *Nat. New Biol.*, 1971; 231, 237–239.
6. ISIS-2 (Second International Study of Infarct Survival) Collaboration Group, Randomised trial of intravenous streptokinase, oral aspirin, both or neither among cases of suspected acute myocardial infarction. *The Lancet*, 1988; 1, 397–402.
7. Julian, D.G., The evolution of the coronary care unit. *Cardiovasc. Res.*, 2001; 51, 621–624.
8. Reynell, P.C. and Reynell M.C., The cost-benefit analysis of a coronary care unit. *Br. Heart J.*, 1972; 34, 897–900.
9. Cretin, S., Cost/Benefit analysis of treatment and prevention of myocardial infarction. *Health Serv. Res.*, 1977; 12, 174–189.
10. Baroldi, G., Acute coronary occlusion as a cause of myocardial infarct and sudden coronary death. *Am. J. Cardiol.*, 1965; 16, 859.
11. Roberts, W.C. and Buja L.M., The frequency and significance of coronary arterial thrombi and other observations in fatal acute myocardial infarction. *Am. J. Med.*, 1972; 52, 425.

12. Armstrong, A., Duncan, B., Oliver, M.F., *et al.*, Natural history of acute coronary heart attacks. *Br. Heart J.*, 1972; 34, 67–80.
13. De Wood, M.A., Spores J., Notske. R., *et al.*, Prevalence of total coronary occlusion during the early hours of transmural myocardial infarction. *N. Eng. J. Med.*, 1980; 303, 897–902.
14. Brooks, N., Intracoronary thrombolysis in acute myocardial infarction. *Br. Heart J.*, 1983; 50, 397–400.

3

The Impact of the Changing Social, Political and Economic Environment on Medical Science

'It's the economy, stupid' was a phrase originally intended by Bill Clinton's campaign team during his 1992 run for the US presidency to focus attention on the economy, which had gone into recession. It has been credited with winning him the election, and even if this seems a bit farfetched, it nevertheless was the right tactic to focus the effort in taking on George H.W. Bush, the incumbent. Bush's approval rating had been high in polls during 1991, soon after the invasion of Iraq, but had fallen sharply the following year as the economy declined. The phrase has since become iconic, not only as a means of emphasising the importance of the economy at all times, but also as a template on which to make almost any point (despite its patronising character). It resonates with the rise in importance of the economy in western cultures during the past two decades. Another political phrase, 'There is no such thing as society,' was attributed to Margaret Thatcher during an interview in 1987. It was intended, not unreasonably, to emphasise self-help as the first port of call for those in difficulty rather than an immediate recourse to the state. However it too has taken on a life of its own as it coincides with what many perceive as a loss of community cohesion as Western cultures become more anonymous and competitive in pursuit of economic growth. One might be tempted to combine the two and say, 'there is no such thing as society, we have become an economy'.

The other two phrases used by Clinton's campaign team in 1992 are often forgotten: 'Change versus more of the same' and 'Don't forget health care'. The latter has certainly become a major political issue in the years that have followed and the three slogans together underline the link between economics and health which increasingly dominates the political agenda in many countries.

Economics and Health: A Two-way Interaction

I was reminded of this when asked by a senior economist whether medical treatment is cost effective. The basis for the question was that although curing a patient reduces the duration and costs of the present illness, this economic benefit is likely to be offset by further expenditure later, which might not have arisen had the patient succumbed to the earlier ailment. The question poses one of the great challenges of the modern era. Life expectancy has increased dramatically in the developed world during the 20th century as living conditions and health care have improved. For example, men born in the US in 1998 could expect to live about 74 years compared with 44 years in 1900.[1] Longer survival means that the age distribution of populations is shifted upwards. This results in a lower working-to-retired ratio and also to further increases in health costs as those who live longer incur more health expenditures in later life. The economic consequences of this are obvious: health care spending has increased in real terms and as a proportion of national budgets during the 20th century. Added to this is a growing awareness of inequalities in health within and between countries. In Britain, death rates* in people under 65 years of age in the 1920s were 90% higher among the poorest than the richest. Rather than declining, this inequality increased during the century, reaching 112% in 1999–2007.[2] Mortality rates vary by as much as sixfold between rich and poor nations globally.[3] These disparities have become a major political issue around the world; there is increasing tension between demand and both the resources available to meet that demand and between different areas of need. Should we be spending more on improving health care in the

---

*Death rate expressed per 1,000 population standardised for age and sex.

developing world and less in rich nations? Should we spend more on prevention and less on treating current illness? To put it more crudely, how much health do we need and how should we measure it? With an aging population and an ample healthy workforce to meet the requirements of our economy, do we really need to spend more? Such questions might seem outrageous to a person with a sick relative, but are bread and butter in health economics, which, as discussed in Chapter 1, now has a major impact on how medicine is practised and how its priorities are set. In the global arena too, economics is having an increasing impact on health care.

Globalisation of Health

Growing awareness of disparities in global health has been a stimulus for increased investment to treat and prevent diseases in developing countries. Public interest is captured in a powerful way by emergencies due to famine, earthquakes and other disasters. Television pictures showing the reality of what is happening on the ground have had a huge global impact. Similarly, efforts to increase awareness of HIV/AIDS and the need for funds to provide drugs to treat it have been extraordinarily successful. Spending rose from $1 billion in 2000 to $11 billion by 2008 in response to unprecedented international lobbying campaigns. Organisations such as the Global Health Council emerged rebranded in the late 1990s as an umbrella for many advocacy groups working to improve global health; the timing of this suggests that the HIV/AIDs campaign was a likely impetus. UNAIDS was founded in 1998 to combat the epidemic and is the only global health programme based on a single disease. The Gates Foundation, set up in 2000, represents an exceptional philanthropic contribution to support poorer nations. The fund provided almost $10 billion in aid of global health up to 2009,[4] providing funds to improve health and to support research for prevention and new treatments. Governments have also committed substantial funding.

Efforts to tackle disparities in global health have been remarkably successful. Two striking examples serve to illustrate this. The substantial increase in the number of individuals treated for HIV infection in poorer countries means that more than 5 million people in low and middle income countries were receiving antiretroviral therapy by the end of 2009 and as a consequence about 14.4 million life years have been gained since 1996.[5] Secondly, a marked reduction in childhood mortality has occurred during the past three decades. Deaths from all causes have reduced 85–93% among children aged between one and four in a range of 50 countries, including many with very low incomes.[6] Mortality among those aged between 15 and 45 also reduced, by about 34% in women and 19% in men between 1970 and 2010.[3] This occurred despite dramatic increases in some regions due to HIV infection, most notably in sub-Saharan Africa where deaths among men and women increased by about 56% and 175% respectively.[3]

The extent to which individual campaigns contribute to these changes and to advances in medical science is more difficult to resolve. Most lobbying focuses on demanding access to treatments at reduced cost and advocating that patent rights be relaxed to allow production of cheaper generic versions of drugs. The reductions in adult and childhood mortality described above are mainly due to reductions in communicable diseases and this trend was well established in the 1960s, decades before the recent attention given to global health and the Millennium Development Goals. It is very likely therefore that these trends would have continued given that the investment in these areas was already in place. Most of the effort to discover new antiviral drugs to treat HIV/AIDs has occurred in developed countries and, since their own populations faced serious risks from the epidemic, it is likely that much of this would have happened anyway. The HIV/AIDS campaigns have been highly successful in focusing the public's attention on the HIV epidemic and can claim to have contributed greatly to the increased availability of antiretroviral drugs for millions of people in poorer countries and to the many lives saved. But it is also increasingly clear that the spread of HIV/AIDS relates to many other cultural and social factors, most notably poverty, lack of education and individual powerlessness, and that investing in these is also needed to curtail the epidemic.[7] Although considerable success has been achieved in delivering treatments for people infected, efforts have been slower to engage at this deeper preventative level. An effective vaccine is still awaited. Lack of education and poverty are major social factors in the spread of HIV/AIDS and will need to be addressed to secure a long-term solution.

Economics of Global Health and Biomedical Science

Following many years of neglect, funding for diseases that occur exclusively or predominantly in the developing world has increased in recent years. Universities around the world have responded by setting up research centres related to global health to capture research contracts to meet the challenge. However many of these appear to be groupings of existing academic units engaged in standard biomedical science, with an added overlay of public health policy and rebranded under a global health banner. Public health scientists[8] with the backing of respected journals[9] have called for open access to research data to improve understanding of global health inequalities. This call appears reasonable and the proposal does include a recognition that scientists in poorer countries should be acknowledged in any subsequent publications. However such a measure loses sight of the fact that many researchers in low-income countries even struggle to pay for access to the scientific literature.

What is needed is a more constructive engagement with low-income countries that builds a lasting scientific infrastructure that will allow scientists in those countries to work as equals with their counterparts from more affluent nations and that leaves a legacy that can help solve future problems locally. Already, concerns about self-interest among Western universities seeking unbalanced collaborations have led to suspicions of a 'new scramble for Africa'.[10] Donations by Western governments and other funders to support research into treatments for diseases in poorer nations sound promising, but if this work is done exclusively in rich countries, even if the products developed are effective, they will be expensive and likely to require further donations to enable low-income countries to purchase them in the future. Since most of these payments will go to those who developed the drugs, little may remain for building a scientific infrastructure in the low-income countries where it is most needed. The search for a vaccine against HIV remains elusive despite huge investment, and what optimism there is arises from discoveries made before the HIV/AIDS epidemic began, namely advances in genetics made in the 1970s which allowed the genome of the virus to be manipulated.[11] The need for ongoing assistance for low-income countries remains and will continue to do so until the epidemic is substantially reversed. Until then funders, governments and campaigners should ask what legacy their investments will leave.

Impact of Lobbying on Biomedical Research

The effects of advocacy and lobbying campaigns on biomedical research are complex. Support for HIV, malaria and tuberculosis amounted to almost 80% of funding provided for research into diseases that afflict low-income countries in 2007, and that excludes spending by governments and industry to combat these diseases in Western countries.[12] In contrast, research into pneumonia and diarrhoeal diseases received only 6% of total funding[12] although they account for 32% more deaths and disability.[13] There are several reasons for this misalignment:

a) The initial effectiveness of advocacy campaigns depends on their ability to capture the attention of the media. This in turn depends on their message going out at sufficient 'volume', by, for example, coordinating events across a number of locations to occur simultaneously, or by providing support for other committed groups to help to spread the call for action. While this can act as a multiplier for the cause and rapidly escalate its place on the public agenda, it also serves to amplify any misalignment between support and need in the objectives of the campaign.

b) For some diseases, the state of science may suggest that a breakthrough is possible. Some funders may wish to channel their investment into research that seems more likely to be productive. While this may be understandable, it raises two issues; firstly, funders may not always be best placed to understand the state of science in a particular area and secondly, scientists may be tempted to oversell the likelihood of an imminent advance given the competition to attract funding.

c) Other funders may decide to invest in poorly-researched areas in the hope of a discovery that will open up a new avenue of research.

d) Yet others may wish to prioritise their investment in proportion to the lack of available treatments or in relation to the lethality of diseases.

Thus, while the generosity of funders is very much to their credit, the basis on which funds are disbursed varies widely and often is not well aligned with need. This misalignment is also reflected in the dominant role that the HIV/AIDS movement has played during the past 25 years. By successfully capturing the attention of people and their governments around the world HIV/AIDS has also had a major impact on priority setting for the distribution of support. But there is now a growing understanding that this focus on HIV/AIDS has excluded other diseases that cause even greater rates of death and disability and support is waning. Evidence of this can be seen in the recent failure of the Global Fund to Fight AIDS, Tuberculosis and Malaria to raise funds for the period 2011 to 2013 to match its spending in previous years; the UN Secretary General announced that only 68% of what had been requested had been made available by donor countries.

While lobbying can be highly effective in motivating the public and governments to take action, particularly in terms of providing prompt assistance for acute emergencies and funds to pay for medicines, it has been less effective as a means to support research according to need in the longer term. For similar reasons, intermittent funding generated by campaigns to support research for specific cures is often out of step with the way science works best. As discussed in Chapter 2, scientific discovery is an unpredictable and often unmanageable process. The highly creative intellectual effort involved does not respond well to direction. In other words, attempts to 'buy' cures have not worked very well in the past, as exemplified by President Nixon's National Cancer Act in 1971.[14] The act has not led to the discovery of a cure for cancer, but the commitment has undoubtedly contributed to many advances in biomedical science, particularly in the field of genetics. The National Cancer Act illustrates again that medical advances and cures are more likely to arise in environments in which creative science is flourishing rather than through research directed to fulfil the well-intended wish lists of funders. The temptation may be to begin by defining the outcome that is most desired, but science works best by defining the first question to ask and leaving the outcome uncertain until the end.

Donor Fatigue

Donor fatigue is a particular concern if it risks interrupting support for long-term needs. It is most likely to arise in response to campaigns that are episodic, related to causes dependent on the media for their fashionable status or motivated by celebrities whose time in the spotlight is often transient. Intermittent fundraising can be very useful for supporting unexpected disasters, but is not appropriate for providing the consistent long-term support needed to combat global endemic diseases or to support biomedical science. It may even hamper scientific progress if established networks are disrupted to meet some short-term need or academic institutions seek to realign their research portfolio to engage transient funding opportunities. It can also be difficult for such campaigns to capture a detailed view of the science involved or the context in which support is needed.

The UN and WHO response to HIV/AIDS was to treat it as a special case, and HIV/AIDS was indeed a new disease and a major global threat. However it was not alone, but rather one of several interdependent epidemics, and the result of this policy affording HIV/AIDS special status was that other major causes of disability, such as TB, malaria, injury and non-communicable diseases, did not receive the attention they needed. Inevitably single-issue activists come to be seen as lacking a balanced view of need and, however deserving the cause they support, risk losing public sympathy and political support. A further danger of single-issue campaigns is that in squeezing out other areas of need, they stimulate other advocacy groups to support those causes deprived, risking a competition for public attention and a wasting of valuable funds. Funders with deep pockets should be able to take a longer-term view and determine their priorities based on carefully defined objectives, evidence of need and likelihood of success. The danger for politicians is the temptation to surf the wave of public interest generated by powerful short-term campaigns and thus divert funds and scientific effort to engage the issues generated by them. This is likely to become a more frequent problem in the future as activists learn how to employ the new communication tactics available on the web to generate an instant media presence. In the case of global health, the intense focus on infectious diseases over the past two decades has undoubtedly contributed to pushing non-communicable diseases down the agenda and it is only now that we seeing a new global effort to redress the balance.[15]

Confidence and Trust in Science

Trust in science became a major issue at the end of the 20th century. This followed decades in which science enjoyed high levels of public confidence, perhaps related to early successes in space exploration, developments in electronics that made computers widely available and advances in medicine that led to a marked increase in longevity. There are several factors that led to an erosion in public trust and confidence in science, but in recent times these seem to have been expressed most powerfully in relation to climate change and the resistance towards genetically modified (GM) food, particularly in the Europe. Originally introduced in 1996, GM plants are genetically modified by modern laboratory techniques to introduce advantages such as resistance to insects or insecticides, or greater yields. Fears that this might have unknown harmful effects on consumers or the environment led to widespread objections, particularly in Europe. In 2010, the controversy over disclosure of climate data at the University of East Anglia (UEA) became the major science issue of the year in the global media and led to warnings that the public was losing trust in science.[16] Understandably, the media played a major role in both these debates; indeed, the Economic and Social Research Council in the UK awarded a grant to study the 'effect of language choices in the debate on Public Trust' in relation to the GM food debate.[17] After the release of the Independent Climate Change Email Review, *The Lancet* commented that science would 'never be the same again'.[9] The speed and intensity of interest in both issues were remarkable and led to concerns that public trust in science was waning. Such intensity is not sustainable given the vagaries of media interest, but in the short term, while campaigns are running, they can lead to a distorted view of public opinion. A reader survey by *Scientific American* and *Nature* conducted months after the 'Climategate' affair suggested that the respondents are more trustful of information received from scientists than from their family and friends, NGOs, citizen groups, journalists, corporations, elected officials or religious authorities. They had greater trust in what scientists say about renewable energy than any other topic polled except evolution and considered them least trustworthy on flu pandemics, drugs for depression, pesticides and GM crops.[18] When asked what technologies caused most concern about unintended consequences, twice as many (47%) stated they were most fearful of nuclear power rather than GM crops (22%). Given the nature of these journals and the fact that the survey was based on their readers, these findings are not surprising.

The UK House of Lords Science and Technology Report into public attitudes towards science talked about a crisis of trust in science, but it could be argued the details of the report suggest a different picture. The House of Lords study, based on a random sample of people, showed that only 4.6% of people were 'most trustful' of government scientists in regard to statements made about bovine spongiform encephalopathy (BSE) and only 0.4% were most trustful of scientists writing in newspapers. These results contrasted sharply with the 42% who were most trustful of independent scientists.[19] A similar pattern emerged for trust regarding nuclear power. In a survey carried out in 15 member states of the European Union in 1999, 89% of people trusted doctors to be truthful, compared with 88% for teachers, 38% for government scientists and 10% for journalists.[17] But again, when asked who would be considered most trusted to tell the truth about pollution, 60% voted for independent scientists compared with 6% for government scientists. A similar picture emerged for BSE; 57% of respondents were most trustful of independent scientists compared with 4% for government scientists. It appears, therefore, that the crisis of trust is not so much focused on science or scientists but on organisations and governments that increasingly use science. The survey results also imply a significant degree of public discernment of events, and resistance to media presentation. Thus, despite the intensity of the short-term reactions reported in the media, public opinion may be harder to shift in the longer term. A comment made in *Nature* about the Climategate affair that 'scientists involved in a street fight should expect some low blows'[16] may be more to the point. Perhaps in time the public may yet reconsider the role the deliberate theft and leaking of UEA emails had in sparking off the affair. Who did it, what was their purpose and what was been done to identify the culprit(s)?

Trust in Medicine and Medical Science

Linked as they are to our most powerful experiences, life and death, it can hardly be surprising that individual and public attitudes to medicine have been varied and become ambivalent over time. Pain and suffering are regarded simply as necessary evils, something to be controlled and avoided in the modern era of analgesia, but this is not always so. Among several religions, pain is considered something to be endured, or at times a blessing, linked to ideas of self-sacrifice and chastity. Some religious groups have condemned certain aspects of medical practice, for example, vaccination, on the grounds that it implants diseased material into a healthy person, and Jehovah's Witnesses are required to refuse blood transfusions, but not organ transplantation.[20] More generally, medicine and religions have had a changing relationship. In ancient times, healing was the prerogative of both priests and physicians. In recent centuries, mainstream religions have been concerned mainly with the soul and medicine with bodily ailments, nevertheless, even in our own time religious healing remains very active. In some instances this involves promoting a general sense of wellbeing or allaying anxiety, but in others healing for illnesses incurable by modern medicine is confidently advertised.

The history of medicine in the pre-scientific era is littered with discarded diseases and diagnoses as well as many useless or harmful treatments.[20] Some were so fanciful or contradictory that they attracted ridicule and satire, as exemplified in George Bernard Shaw's, *The Doctor's Dilemma*. Later in the 20th century, medicine would find its most powerful and strident critics. The harshest of these was Ivan Illich, who postulated that medicine was part of a capital-intensive production system that treated patients as commodities. The result, he believed, was that people were deprived of the natural experience of pain, illness and death. He further argued that medicine contributed nothing to mortality rates and that iatrogenic illness is now a major threat to human health. His book, *Medical Nemesis*,[21] published in 1974, has been highly influential among policy makers and social scientists in arguing for a redistribution of investment away from medicine. Public health activists have been ambivalent about his views; some have supported and repeated his arguments that acute medical interventions have little to offer in advancing health, but others have been irritated by Illich's inclusion of public health medicine in his depiction of what he called a destructive medical industry.

Two other books published in the 1970s have also proven to be highly influential in shaping health care policy during the past three decades.

In *The Role of Medicine; Dream, Mirage or Nemesis*, Thomas McKeown concluded that reductions in human mortality from 1700 to 1930 were the result of improved economic and social conditions and that medical advances contributed little.[22] A.L. Cochrane's book *Effectiveness and Efficiency; Random Reflections on Health Services*[23] criticised the medical profession for not producing reliable evidence on which to base practice and championed randomised controlled clinical trials. Although the two authors draw quite different conclusions, they are frequently cited together as background support in comments and arguments that are critical of interventional medicine as inefficient and wasteful and whose practitioners are too powerful and in favour of diverting investment and power towards social intervention and public health. Inaccuracies in McKeown's analysis and interpretation of mortality data have led some to question his objectivity, and to regard his thesis as discredited.[24] Nevertheless his work continues to be influential, particularly in the fields of social science and public health. Cochrane continues to be widely revered and defended as a leader who gave us evidence-based medicine (EBM).[25] However his most influential work[23] was itself purely rhetorical and anecdotal, and his actual experience of randomised controlled clinical trials was minimal. Indeed Cochrane's most striking success may have been in capturing the agenda for setting the direction of medicine over the past three decades based around the idea of EBM; essentially a propaganda coup which has been highly effective in leveraging power towards public health and social medicine and away from what he regarded as wasteful and inefficient, that is, clinical medicine. A strident attack on the EBM movement[26] was met with derision by some media commentators[25] but the essential criticisms of its rhetorical and political methods and its tendency to accumulate power for itself need to be explored.[27] In my own field, Cochrane's premature antagonism towards coronary care units and his apparent unwillingness to acknowledge their contributions to understanding the natural history and pathology of coronary disease are worrying signs of selective enthusiasm. This also exemplifies the inherent dangers, which a narrow interpretation of EBM holds for medical science, for much of what is done in science is based on hypothesis rather than evidence. I have no doubt that Cochrane, or Archie, as he was better known to his many friends, was a charming and much-loved man, however I am doubtful that he would have been comfortable with the manner in which the EBM movement has been built around an apparent cult of personality.[28] Neither do I suspect his distinctly left-wing sensibilities would have left him entirely happy to have a centre named after him that is funded by a government department pursuing a neoliberal agenda.

In recent years medicine has also faced the exposure of medical scandals in the media, and there have been widespread fears in the medical community of plummeting public confidence as a result. In the UK there was the case of GP Harold Shipman, convicted of multiple murders in 2000, and the failures at the Bristol Royal Infirmary and Alder Hey Hospital. Doctors were urged to confess their mistakes by the National Patient Safety Agency so that the root causes of 'litanies of failure' could be addressed.[29] In the US the profession also feels beleaguered by claims that public trust has been eroded because of increasing specialisation, conflicts of interest and commercial links, with doctors often owning for-profit clinical facilities. The solution proposed is a 'Marshall Plan' to rebuild public confidence[30] by removing financial pressures on medical students and addressing shortages of doctors in primary care by forgiving the student debt of junior doctors in exchange for working in poorly-serviced areas. In the UK a report calling for a new compact between the profession, patients and government[31] was well received, but initial hopes of a new, depoliticised NHS faded rapidly as the service soon became the centre of yet another round of reforms and intense political activity.

Individual doctors seem to have stood back from much of this. One consequence has been that few of them have been willing to take on managerial roles in the service.[32,33] There is also evidence that they have less confidence in some of their leaders and have disengaged from medical politics. In a letter to its fellows, the Royal College of Physicians in London warned that it was wasting money because only 26% of the 14,000 ballot papers for its 2010 presidential election were returned. The suggestion that such low participation may reflect a dull election procedure or that doctors are too busy being good doctors seems unlikely to be responsible since the election has always been dull and doctors have always been busy. A more likely explanation is that fellows have felt that the College has sought to align itself too closely with the Department of Health at a time when doctors have felt under siege by it. Comments from past presidents about 'not banging the table' at the Department of Health to avoid 'not being invited back' are likely to have been regarded as post hoc apologetics. This misalignment between leaders and practicing doctors came to a head when the chairman of the British Medical Association (BMA) had to resign in 2007 over a letter he and a former president of the Royal College of Physicians wrote to *The Times* newspaper in support of the Chief Medical Officer's role in what turned out to be a disastrous scheme for recruiting junior doctors.[34] Some even feel that the government conspired to discredit doctors before the public.[35] I am reminded of the advice given by a rising star in medical politics in 1992 who, when asked by an administrator colleague what to do about doctors who don't do what you want them to do, replied 'you should make an example of a few of them.' An aggressive posture and confidence has certainly served some administrators well in subsequent years of climbing the greasy poll of medical politics.

Despite all of the upheavals and reforms of health care over the past two decades, it appears that the public continues to hold doctors in high regard. A series of MORI polls conducted for the BMA between 1983 and 2005 has repeatedly shown that doctors enjoy consistently high levels of public trust; indeed levels that are several times greater than politicians or journalists, and this has remained undented over the years.[36] Thus, individual doctors and scientists appear to have weathered challenges to the trust in which they are held by the public. They nevertheless face changing fortunes generated by fashions and politics. This has important implications for scientists and the relationships they form with agencies that need scientific advice. This was highlighted in 2009 when the UK Home Secretary sacked Professor David Nutt, head of the Advisory Council on Drug Misuse, for expressing views contrary to government policy. Nutt's comments were made while giving a scientific paper to an academic body and his sacking caused an outcry within the scientific community.[37] It seems clear that scientific advice can only be of use so long as it is independent and that advice which is tailored to conform to government policy is little more than propaganda. The government's response to the Nutt affair was to promise new guidance that would respect the independence of scientific advice, but the initial draft called for scientific advisors and ministers to 'work together to reach a shared position, and neither should act to undermine mutual trust', which again brought protests from scientists.[38] That there should be tension between governments and scientists is not surprising or new. Similar concerns have been expressed in many countries.[39,40] Preserving their independence is crucial for scientists; not only to ensure that the advice they give is of value, but also because their integrity and public regard depend on it. This is certain to be tested more and more in the future as academic institutions become more financially dependent on government and industry. Fields that impinge on government policy are particularly vulnerable. Health policy is one, but economics, social sciences and nuclear power will also be important.

On an international level, confidence in what medical science can achieve appears to be being questioned in some important areas. For example, a paper published by the WHO in 2004, and widely referenced since, set out what it saw as the priority needs for new medicines.[41] Despite the predominant impact of cardiovascular disease on global health, which is predicted to increase in the developing world,[42] the authors felt that apart from a polypill to combine preventive medicines and treatment for acute stroke, no cardiovascular diseases merited priority. In a similar vein, the potential contribution that medical science can make seems to be disregarded by some who seek to reform medical education with a view to meeting the challenge of global health inequalities.[43] There appears to be a lack of vision or confidence or both regarding what biomedical science can achieve.

This view of medicine — that the time comes when the science has been done and the laboratory apparatus can be decommissioned to allow clinicians to focus more efficiently on the delivery of care — is deeply flawed for two reasons. Firstly, there are countless new discoveries to be made in the future that will transform how medicine is practised if we have the vision and confidence to pursue them. Secondly, the capacity to do science is one of our greatest assets and takes generations to establish. To discard it in the name of efficiency would be calamitous and could not be easily reversed. As for the view that there are no priorities left for cardiovascular medicine other than a polypill and treatment for acute stroke,[41] one common example may serve to illustrate its short sightedness. High blood pressure is a major cause of death and disability in the developing world. At present understanding of its cause remains obscure and the only effective treatment is lifelong medication for the vast majority of people, which on a global scale is surely daunting. And yet, if the causes of hypertension could be unravelled, prevention might well be possible. But we are misled into thinking we understand hypertension because blood pressure can be measured using a sphygmomanometer and, as treatments are available, nothing further needs to be done. But one day its pathophysiology will be understood and hypertension will be preventable. As with so many developments in the past, its achievement may be sparked by a serendipitous observation by a curious and stubborn mind, probably working far removed from what is fashionable and swimming against the tide of contemporary interests.

The dangers for biomedical science in the 21st century therefore may not so much result from a lack of trust among the public, but rather a loss of vision and understanding among policy makers and governments about how science works and what it can achieve. In their desperation to achieve reform of health care policy, a long tradition of clinical science has already been seriously damaged. There appears to be a growing sense among governments and research funders that scientific discoveries can be bought off the shelf on demand. This may in part relate to the success of technological applications such as the Human Genome Project and the misconception that original science can be successfully managed in a similar way. Some funders now regard their role as commissioners of research; their function being to develop a vision of what science needs to do in a particular area to achieve success as if it can then be purchased by tender and managed from above by a committee far removed from the laboratory bench. But ideas come from individuals, not committees, and the best ideas come from those doing the science. In many ways, this managerial approach harks back to the classic 'scientific' management techniques introduced into industry during the 20th century to improve the efficiency of repetitive tasks. But such direction has no place in creative work such as original science, where continual questioning is a necessity rather than a hindrance to efficiency. Such management loses sight of, and fails to harness, the most valuable assets that make science work: individual human curiosity and creativity. As the Nobel Prize winner Ahmed Zewail put it, 'history teaches us the value of free scientific inquisitiveness'.[44] The challenge facing medical science is to maintain that culture of original enquiry and freedom to explore new avenues which proved so effective during the 20th century. This may not be an easy message to convey in an era dominated by short-term economic perspectives, but is one which leaders of medicine must have the courage to take forward to ensure that the environment of biomedical science they inherited is preserved for their successors.

Summary and Conclusions

The social and political environment in which medical science exists has changed radically in the past three decades. The rising cost of health care has focused an economic lens with a new set of priorities on all of medical science's activities, which has undermined many of its traditional strengths. We live much longer than previously and incur greater health expenditure as a result. Reforms of health care delivery are pursued with an intensity that borders on desperation and has degraded the culture of medical science.

The horizon of health has also widened dramatically in line with economic globalisation, as powerfully illustrated by the HIV/AIDs pandemic. Global health has become a major social and political issue and has led to unprecedented investment by governments and private donors in public health at a global level. This has been remarkably successful in funding treatment for victims of HIV/AIDs, but other areas of need, including some with greater potential to cause death and disability, have been neglected. The emotive power of health campaigns can be highly effective in driving the political agenda, but they lack objectivity in relation to overall priorities for health and medical science.

Public trust in science and medicine has also been questioned in recent years, but surveys of public opinion have consistently shown that this relates more to industrial uses of science and to the opinions expressed by scientists who work for industry or governments. In contrast, independent scientists continue to enjoy higher levels of trust. This also is the case for medicine and medical science. The pharmaceutical industry suffers from low levels of public trust, whereas doctors continue to be held in high regard.

Medical science in the 21ˢᵗ century faces a much harsher social and political environment than previously. Despite its proven capacity to provide solutions for health needs and challenges, it often fails to find a place among the short-term economic priorities of health policy makers in their search for efficiency. Despite this, immense health challenges remain and these will, in time, bring new economic challenges into focus, which I believe will force a reversal of the present involution. Meanwhile it is essential to retain the embers of the culture we inherited so that our successors can rekindle its flame.

References

1. Smith, D.W. and Bradshaw, B.S., Annual mortality report: life expectancy increase. *Demography*, 2006; 43, 647–657.
2. Thomas, B., Dorling D. and Smith, G.D., Inequalities in premature mortality in Britain: observational study from 1921 to 2007. *BMJ*, 2010; 341, c3639.
3. Rajaratnam, J.K., Marcus, J.R., Levin-Rector, A., *et al.*, Worldwide mortality in men and women aged 15–59 years from 1970 to 2010: a systematic analysis. *The Lancet*, 2010; 375, 1704–1720.
4. Bill & Melinda Gates Foundation, Global health: strategy overview. September 2010. http://www.gatesfoundation.org/global-health/Documents/global-health-strategy-overview.pdf. Accessed 4 July 2012.
5. UNAIDS, Global report: UNAIDS report on the global AIDS epidemic. 2010. http://www.unaids.org/globalreport/Global_report.htm. Accessed 4 July 2012.
6. Viner, R.M., Coffey, C., Mathers, C., *et al.*, 50-year mortality trends in children and young people: a study of 50 low-income, middle-income, and high-income countries. *The Lancet*, 2011; 377, 1162–1174.
7. Muchini, B., Benedikt, C., Gregson, S., *et al.*, Local perceptions of forms, timing and causes of behaviour change in response to the AIDS epidemic in Zimbabwe. *AIDS behav.*, 2011; 15, 487–498.
8. Walport, M. and Brest, P., Sharing research data to improve public heath. *The Lancet*, 2011; 377, 537–539.
9. Horton, R., Science will never be the same again. *The Lancet*, 2010; 376, 143–144.
10. Crane, J., Scrambling for Africa? Universities and global health. *The Lancet*, 2011; 377, 1388–1389.

11. McCullers, J.A. and Dunn, J.D., Advances in vaccine technology and their impact on managed care. *Pharmacy and Therapeutics*, 2008; 33, 35–41.
12. Moran, M., Guzman, J., Ropars, A.L., *et al.*, Neglected disease research and development: how much are we really spending? *PLoS Medicine*, 2009; 6, 0137–0146.
13. WHO, Global burden of disease. 2004 update. http://www.who.int/healthinfo/global_burden_disease/GBD_report_2004update_full.pdf. Accessed 5 July 2012.
14. National Cancer Act of 1971. http://www.dtp.nci.nih.gov/timeline/noflash/milestones/M4_Nixon.htm. Accessed 5 July 2012.
15. Beaglehole, R., Bonita, R., Horton, R., *et al.*, Priority actions for the non-communicable disease crisis. *The Lancet*, 2011; 377, 1438–1447.
16. Closing the climategate. *Nature*, 2010; 468, 345.
17. Cook, G., Pieri, E. and Robbins, P., The discourse of the GM food debate: how language choices affect public trust. Economic and Social Research Council grant report, January 2004. http://www.esrc.ac.uk/my-esrc/grants/RES-000-22-0132/outputs/Read/909488e6-4f21-4e1b-ab68-e65d44303881. Accessed 15 August 2012.
18. In science we trust. *Scientific American*, October 2010; 56–59.
19. House of Lords Science and Technology Committee, Third report. Febuary 2000. http://www.publications.parliament.uk/pa/ld199900/ldselect/ldsctech/38/3816.htm. Accessed 5 July 2012.
20. Porter, R., What is disease? in *The Cambridge Illustrated History of Medicine*, Ed. by Porter, R., Cambridge University Press, Cambridge, 1996. p. 82-117.
21. Illich, I., *Medical Nemesis*. Calder and Boyers, London, 1974.
22. McKeown, T., *The Role of Medicine: Dream, Mirage or Nemesis?* Nuffield Provincial Hospitals Trust, London, 1976.
23. Cochrane, A.L., *Effectiveness and Efficiency: Random Reflections on Health Services*. Nuffield Provincial Hospitals Trust, London, 1972.
24. Colgrove, J., The McKeown thesis: a historical controversy and its enduring influence. *Am. J. Public Health*, 2002; 92, 725–729.
25. Goldacre, B., Bad science. *The Guardian*, 19 August 2006. http://www.bad-science.net/2006/08/archie-cochrane-fascist/. Accessed 5 July 2012.
26. Holmes, D., Murray, S.J., Perron, A., *et al.*, Deconstructing the evidence-based discourse in health sciences: truth, power and fascism. *Int. J. Evid. Based Healthc.*, 2006; 4, 180–186.

27. Healy, B., Who says what's best? *US News and World Report*, 3 September 2006. http://www.usnews.com/usnews/health/articles/060903/11healy.htm. Accessed 5 July 2012.
28. Archie Cochrane: the name behind the Cochrane Collaboration. The Cochrane Collaboration website. http://www.cochrane.org/about-us/history/archie-cochrane. Accessed 5 July 2012.
29. Senior doctors admit mistakes in campaign for more open culture. *BMJ*, 2005; 331, 595.
30. Shomaker, T.S., The 'Medical Marshall Plan': rebuilding public trust in American medicine. *Acad. Med.*, 2010; 85, 1680.
31. Ham, C. and Alberti, K.G.M.M., The medical profession, the public, and the government. *BMJ*, 2002; 324, 838.
32. Morrison, P.E., Heineke, J., Why do health care practitioners resist quality management? *Qual. Prog.*, 1992; 25(4), 51–55.
33. Shekelle, P.G., Why don't physicians enthusiastically support quality improvement programmes? *Qual. Saf. Health Care*, 2002; 11, 6.
34. BMA chairman resigns over MTAS letter to the Times. *BMJ*, 2007; 334, 1074–1075.
35. Is the BMJ fit for purpose? *BMJ*, 2007; 335, 318.
36. Ford, J., Public trust in doctors undented. *BMJ*, 2007; 335, 465.
37. Gossop, M. and Hall, W., Clashes between the government and its expert advisors. *BMJ*, 2009; 339, 1095–1096.
38. Dyer, C., Scientists protest against proposals on advisory group membership. *BMJ*, 2010; 340, 384. Accessed 5 July 2012.
39. The A to Z guide to political interference in science. Union of Concerned Scientists website. http://www.ucsusa.org/scientific_integrity/abuses_of_science/a-to-z-guide-to-political.html. Accessed 5 July 2012.
40. Harding, L., Russia's scientists shun Putin's embrace. *The Guardian*, 31 March 2007. http://www.guardian.co.uk/world/2007/mar/31/russia.luke-harding? INTCMP=SRCH. Accessed 5 July 2012.
41. Kaplan, W. and Laing, R., Priority medicines for Europe and the world. November 2004. http://whqlibdoc.who.int/hq/2004/WHO_EDM_PAR_2004.7.pdf. Accessed 5 July 2012.
42. Lopez, A.D, Mathers, C.D., Ezzati, M., *et al.*, Global and regional burden of disease and risk factors, 2001: systematic analysis of population health data. *The Lancet*, 2007; 367, 1747–1757.

43. Frenk, J., Chen, L., Bhutta, Z.A., *et al.*, Health professionals for a new century: transforming education to strengthen health systems in an interdependent world. *The Lancet*, 2010; 376, 1923.
44. Zewail, A., Curiouser and curiouser: managing discovery making. *Nature*, 2010; 468, 347.

4

Fraud in Biomedical Science

Fraud in science has hit the headlines in recent decades. The intense interest that has surrounded such news is a measure of how unexpected it appears to have been. Media presentations tend to favour revelations of wrongdoing among the most trusted in society. It fits well with the media hunger for stories about the rise and fall of people, institutions and organisations, and the higher the rise or the deeper the fall, the greater the interest. Several successful books on the topic have been published; the list of titles available suggests a lucrative market. Newspaper science editors have been busy filtering the large amount of material that arrives on their desks; one reported receiving 158 items, representing 500,000 words, during four days in 1995.[1]

Science journals too have been busy; the latest cases are of great interest to scientists, as are reviews of old ones. Journal editors have been involved in discussions about their own role in the matter and on the strengths and weakness of peer review, on which they rely for selecting worthy articles to print. The results of their deliberations are followed closely by scientists as well as by the general media. Claims of conspiracies of silence and attempted cover-ups by colleagues and institutions add an element of spice to the mix and enhance copy value further. The idea of the lone investigator pursuing a trail of intrigue against a corrupt establishment has all the ingredients of a hero and villain story to make for excellent reading, particularly when the writer is uncovering something previously unknown.

How Prevalent is Fraud in Science?

By its nature scientific misconduct involves deception and therefore will not usually be obvious. Are the well-publicised cases we learn about the result of just a few bad apples or are they the tip of an iceberg? Obtaining reliable information is difficult and the evidence available relies on survey material. The most recent meta-analysis[2] identified 18 surveys carried out between 1988 and 2005, which used random selections of scientists and were judged to be of good quality. Fraud in these studies was defined as fabrication or falsification of data or the deliberate concealment of data in a manner that would distort scientific knowledge.

Seven surveys which asked if the respondents had ever fabricated or falsified research data or altered results to improve outcome, drew affirmative replies from an average of 2.59% of respondents. If the question was limited to fabrication or falsification, as it was in four surveys, an average of 1.06% of respondents replied 'yes'. Knowledge of a colleague who had fabricated or falsified research data or altered results to improve an outcome[2] was reported by 14.12%. Over the 17 years during which the studies were carried out, the rate of self-reports declined but reports of colleagues' misdeeds did not. Whether this reflects an actual reduction in misconduct in response to better education or less willingness to admit it is unclear. Reports of misconduct were more frequent among medical scientists than in other fields. This might reflect a greater problem among such scientists; alternatively it may be due to a greater willingness to admit fraud. The difference between self-reports and reports of colleagues' misconduct seems striking and larger than might be expected. Under-reporting of personal misconduct or inaccurate knowledge of colleagues' deeds (e.g., unsubstantiated rumour) are both possible, but cannot be confirmed. Similarly, the decline in self-reports of misconduct may not be reliable, particularly as reports of colleagues' misdeeds remained unchanged. In a broader historical perspective, these findings are also complicated by changes in research methods. The introduction of statistics has given a better understanding of optimal study design; we know much more about the importance of sample size, random selection and various forms of bias than in centuries past and so the design of research protocols employed in the past cannot be expected to conform to current standards.

Despite its inherent limitations, the survey approach is probably the best available to capture some idea of the prevalence of fraud in science. This study and its predecessors also found evidence of misconduct in all of the countries studied and in all fields of study. The question arises as to whether this is a new phenomenon or a recent exposure of something that has been longstanding but hidden. Fraud is always bad, but if what we are seeing is new, it indicates a new threat to science and the benefits it produces. Bad science distorts knowledge, diverts effort and stalls or reverses progress.

Although it may be difficult to derive an accurate picture about changing prevalence over time, claims that misconduct in science is new, or that it has arisen sporadically since the 1960s,[3] are certainly not correct. The history of fraud in academia is a long one and is probably as old as human nature itself. It seems to me that this should not come as a great surprise, bearing in mind the history of humanity with all its wonders and weaknesses. Perhaps the earliest example of data manipulation relates to long held suspicions, by Newton among others, that Ptolemy, who lived in the 2nd century AD, was less than candid in his derivation of his astronomical tables in the *Almagest*; these are suspected to have been based on reiterative computation rather than on observations over 800 years, as he claimed.[4]

Research Fraud

Fraud, misconduct or incompetence may arise at any point in the scientific process and can take several forms (Box 4.1). During the experimental stage, fraud may be perpetrated by fabricating or falsifying results to give

---

Box 4.1

Types of Fraud in Science

- Fabrication of data
- Falsification of data
- Omission of data
- Deliberate bias of experiments

a favoured end point. Alternatively, some results may be deliberately omitted for the same reason. In addition, results could be distorted by an experiment that had been deliberately designed to give a favoured result. All have the ability to distort the truth and deflect scientific effort, and all are serious fraud.

Fraud and Misconduct During Publication

Misconduct can also be carried out during the preparation of research or later when it is published (Box 4.2). The most frequent form is plagiarism, in which sections of text or entire articles are copied verbatim. This may not seriously distort the body of scientific knowledge, but it is at best wasteful of resources devoted to publication as well as reviewers' and researchers' time. Plagiarism may also occur if text or ideas are copied and used in preparing grant applications. This may be more difficult to detect, as the entire grant application process is confidential. The consequences may be serious however if funds are awarded to applicants who lack the ability to undertake the work. At best funding is wasted, at worst

Box 4.2

Types of Publication Misconduct

- Plagiarism
- Conflicts of interest
- Breaching confidentiality
- Guest authorship
- Ghost authorship
- Theft of concepts or ideas

Possible Perpetrators

- Journal owners
- Editors
- Authors
- Peer reviewers

incompetent or fraudulent results may be produced. A more worrying and insidious aspect is the wider use of plagiarism by students to complete school and college exercises due to the vast amount of material available on the internet. Apart from the fact that little knowledge is gained in the process, this practice introduces students to deceit, which is exactly the wrong way to inculcate the value of integrity.

Conflicts of interest arise when a personal interest may interfere with the proper functioning of the publication process. Journal owners and editors could try to influence editorial policy for commercial or other reasons. Authors may have a personal interest in the results they are seeking to publish. Reviewers, who are selected because of their experience in the same field, might be tempted to give an adverse review of a competitor's work, or an editor could select reviewers known for destructive or constructive reports in order to influence the selection process.

Manuscripts submitted for publication are regarded as confidential until published. Editors or reviewers might be tempted to breach this confidentiality for a variety of reasons. A dishonest reviewer could write an adverse report and then use the ideas or concepts in that report to further his or her own research and publications. More seriously, some clinical trials may contain information that could have a major impact (positive or negative) on the fortunes of a company involved in the research. Such knowledge is privileged and it is forbidden to use it for share-trading purposes in order to prevent distorting the fair operation of markets.

Guest authorship refers to a colleague who is invited to be an author on a paper, but who has not made a significant contribution to it. This can arise if a senior colleague who has been helpful is invited out of a sense of courtesy, or alternatively it might occur if a scientist with a known reputation is invited to be an author in order to add credibility. Both are wrong in principal and in practice.

Ghost authorship occurs when a professional writer is engaged to write a paper which does not acknowledge his or her contribution when published. This might occur when a paper reporting a large clinical trial involving many collaborators is drafted by a professional writer who had no involvement with the study itself. Provided the final draft of the paper is adequately scrutinised, and can be defended by the authors, such a practice may be acceptable. Alternatively, if an article reviewing commercially sensitive areas of clinical management is written by a professional writer, but is then published under the name of a known authority in the field who is paid for it, there is a serious risk of conflict of interest.

When the Wrong Result is Not Fraud

One of the problems in dealing with fraud in science is the need to distinguish between it and science that produces a wrong answer, but without the intention to deceive. This may happen for several reasons. Building theories or hypotheses is a critical step in science. Research projects usually begin with scientists making a reasoned judgment as to the most likely answer to a question based on his or her knowledge and understanding of the field. Known as hypothesis generation, this is essentially a creative process. Most scientific research involves experiments to prove whether such hypotheses are true or false. When a hypothesis is proven to be false or wrong, the result is still constructive because it helps to direct future work. If an experiment produces a result which is later shown to be wrong, possibly due to some previously unknown interference in the experiment, the result, although incorrect, is not fraudulent. If the scientists are misled by an experiment because it was poorly designed, the result may also be wrong, but in this case it is due to incompetence and not necessarily fraud. If a scientist were to design an experiment in such a way as to give an answer he or she favoured, the result would be both wrong and fraudulent. It is important to understand these distinctions because they need to be managed differently; for example, education may be appropriate in some cases, while others may call for some form of punishment, or both.

The types of fraud outlined above appear straightforward in principal but their execution in practice is far more complex, and understanding their motivation even more so. This needs to be considered when developing effective means for the detection and prevention of such frauds. I have chosen from several fields of science some examples of misconduct and hoaxes from the recent and distant past which I hope will help to illustrate the variety and complexity of fraud.

Case Histories

Forgery

The French mathematician Michel Chasles published thousands of letters between 1861 and 1869, which he had unwittingly purchased from Denis Vrain-Lucas, a forger and writer of remarkable talent. These included letters purportedly written by Isaac Newton, Blaise Pascal and Robert Boyle. When, based on the letters, Chasles claimed in 1867 that Pascal had discovered the law of gravity before Newton, suspicions were raised. Debate continued for two years until Vrain-Lucas was eventually convicted of forgery and imprisoned. After his release in 1872, Vrain-Lucas went on to other deceptions that attracted further prison terms. It seems remarkable now that the forger had managed to carry on the deception for so long in light of his extraordinary output, which included letters from such eminent historical figures as Mary Magdalene, Cleopatra, Judas Iscariot, Pontius Pilate, Joan of Arc and Cicero. A deception of such naiveté and extravagance might suggest a personality disorder, and his letter to Chasles in 1871, written during his first period in prison and translated by historian Ken Alder in 2004,[5] gives an extraordinary insight into the mind and intellect of the forger. A combination of such excellence in penmanship and ability for self-deception goes a long way to explain his behaviour and also perhaps his ability to deceive others. One is almost left regretting what such a mind might have achieved had it been directed to honest toil.

Falsified Evidence: When a Hoax is Fraud

The Piltdown Man affair was one of the most notorious frauds of the 20th century, misleading many for a long time. Described by some as a 'hoax', it refers to the find of a collection of bone fragments at Piltdown, England. These were claimed to be from the skull of an early human and to represent an evolutionary 'missing link' between modern humans and apes. The original finder, Charles Dawson, a solicitor and antiquarian, presented the bone fragments to his collaborator, Arthur Smith Woodward, at the geological department of the British Museum. The material was published in great detail in 1913[6] but appeared anonymously in the *British*

Medical Journal (*BMJ*) in 1912.[7] The evidence was controversial from the outset. Arthur Keith at the Royal College of Surgeons (and possibly the pen behind the *BMJ* articles) challenged the proposed reconstruction of the fragments, suggesting instead that they resembled a modern human, although he played this down two decades later when he unveiled a memorial to the find at Piltdown in 1938.[8] Other scientists with backgrounds in palaeontology and biology also challenged the claims that the Piltdown Man represented a 'missing link', including one accurate description of the fragments as those of a modern human cranium and orang-utan jaw with filed-down teeth.[9]

The debate continues as to who the perpetrators of this fraud were and what role each might have played, whether forger, pitiable dupe or accomplice. A unique aspect of the Piltdown case is that there is convincing evidence of deliberate tampering with the physical evidence of the find; the teeth fragments were deliberately filed down to give them an appearance more compatible with that of an ancient hominid. The word 'hoax' does not go far enough to describe this incident; tampering with the evidence on which scientific conclusions are based is straightforward fraud. The truth finally emerged in 1953 when it was confirmed that the bone fragments consisted of an orang-utan jaw which had been altered and a human skull.[10] It is clear that the Piltdown affair never had much credibility for a few well-informed scientists, but it certainly distracted many and diverted much effort from pursuing the correct path to unravelling the story of human evolution.

When Fraud is Used to Perpetrate a Hoax

Deliberate fraud can also be committed as an intended hoax. In 2010, Professor John McLachlan submitted an abstract for a presentation at a conference on integrative medicine claiming to have discovered that the human body is represented on the buttocks in a manner that responds to stimuli such as acupuncture. The scientific committee accepted his submission. However the abstract was a fiction intended to test whether the conference organisers would accept such claims at face value, question them or seek any clarification. He declined the invitation to attend the conference, but did publish his account in the Christmas edition of the

BMJ,[11] which is generally given over to articles containing an element of humour. The conference organisers were understandably upset at what they considered to be his deceitful actions. But the intention was clearly to test the scientific rigour of the conference by submitting a fictional abstract that would be considered nonsense by any rational observer. For a hoax to succeed the deception must be revealed in time, which is the case here; there was no intention of concealment or of perpetuating the affair as would be the case with intended fraud.

Self-deception

The discovery of N-rays by René Blondlot at the beginning of the 20th century was quickly followed by confirmation of their existence by many other scientists. Initially N-rays were believed to be additional rays produced by X-ray tubes, but later many other sources, such as the Sun and heated metals, were claimed to produce them. Their detection depended on measuring the brightness of faint objects by direct observation, and so would have been subject to variations in visual sensitivity. Normal adaptability of the human eye to varying light conditions made accurate measurement very difficult or impossible. A fundamental requirement for scientific accuracy is that measurements should be objective, that is, independent of the observer, using stable and validated methods. Furthermore, the observer should be unaware of the condition being tested to avoid any risk of unconscious bias. The 'discovery' of N-rays and the large number of confirmations that followed appear to have fallen foul of these errors. Controversy inevitably arose as many papers continued to be published 'confirming' the existence of N-rays, while other scientists could find no evidence of them. Blondlot invited physicist R.W. Wood to visit his laboratory in 1904 to observe experiments, during which Wood became convinced that the observations being made were entirely subjective and were not reproducible in a manner that he could observe. Further work in the field declined rapidly after a report on Wood's observations was published in *Nature*.[12] In it, he remarked that his colleagues were convinced of what they could see and in view of the fact that so many others also reported being able to observe the changes in light intensity on which the results depended, it seems more likely that the affair was due to poor experimental control and lack of objectivity in their design. In other words, the N-ray case was more likely an example of poor science than of science fraud.

On the Fringes of Science

Reports of radiation emitted by dividing cells, known as mitogenetic rays, by Alexander Gurwitsch in 1923 were also confirmed by many scientists, while others failed to detect any evidence of them. Controversy followed, in which Gurwitsch had many supporters and detractors. The clearly-written and detailed paper by Egon Lorenz in 1934,[13] in which no radiation was detected, ended the affair for Western science. However, Gurwitsch continued to flourish in the Soviet sphere, winning the Stalin Prize for his discovery in 1941. In addition, papers continue to appear from time to time discussing aspects of mitogenetic radiation on the fringes of science and in the field that is commonly referred to as alternative healing.

Lack of Peer Scrutiny

In the field of physics, the 'cold fusion' affair is perhaps the most famous case of the 20th century. Martin Fleischmann and Stanley Pons reported an experiment in 1989 claiming that electrolysis of heavy water (water in which hydrogen is replaced by its stable isotope deuterium) on a palladium electrode resulted in an excess production of heat, which they believed could only have come from a nuclear reaction.[14] By announcing their findings to the media before formal publication, 'cold fusion' became a global headline. However it soon became clear that their findings could not be reliably replicated. The case also had some unique features. The scientists involved were of high calibre, with distinguished and respected records, and they were willing to contribute to a formal review of their results. What went wrong in this case was the announcement of their 'discovery' to the media before their work had gone through a normal peer review process. Had this not occurred, it is very likely that flaws in their work would have been revealed, publication delayed or modified, and the media furore dampened. A backdrop of competition to be first out with the news and for patent rights may have contributed to the pair breaking the normal means of communicating scientific results. It is quite possible that the experiments reported by Fleischmann and Pons were performed faithfully, but with some weakness that prevented others from repeating them, meaning the pair's actions were not fraudulent in themselves. However key elements of the science process are objectivity and scepticism and these rely on scrutiny by other experienced scientists. In this case, careful reviews of work did not occur until several years after that press announcement.

False Allegations of Fraud

Gregor Mendel has been hailed as the father of modern genetics, but he has also been accused of producing results that were too good to be true. The allegations arose after the significance of his work was rediscovered in the early 20th century and were based on the application of new statistical methods.[15] The context is that a scientific dispute occurred in the first two decades of the 20th century between those who supported Mendel's genetic model of inheritance and those who favoured a phenotype approach. But Mendel's findings have been replicated by later workers and are clearly true. Confirmation bias has been suggested to explain what has been claimed to be his unexpected precision. This might have occurred if he had observed a result close to what he anticipated and then continued to collect data until the results matched it more closely. However, recent careful analysis of Mendel's paper and of Ronald Fisher's criticism of it[15] has shown that the allegations were in fact unfounded.[16]

Convicted by Whisper and Repetition of False Allegations

In 1923 Robert Millikan was honoured with a Nobel Prize for his work on measuring the charge on electrons. He has since been accused of manipulating his data by selecting only those findings that fitted his theory and discarding the rest.[17] The background to this is that Gerald Holton, a science historian, reviewed Millikan's laboratory notebooks and noticed some differences between Millikan's published work and what the notebooks contained. Holton did not accuse Millikan of any wrongdoing, but his publication, 25 years after Millikan's death, was enough to allow journalists William Broad and Nicholas Wade to dispatch Millikan's reputation in their 1983 book *Betrayers of Truth: Fraud and Deceit in the Halls of Science*. Uncritical repetition of their allegations has perpetuated the assault on Millikan's reputation.

False Allegations are no Better than Research Fraud

As in Mendel's case, Millikan was correct in his findings, which are no longer disputed. The basis for Holton's remarks was that, in his 1913 paper, Millikan stated that his findings were derived from all data collected over a 60-day period, whereas his notebooks contain many more observations. On the face of it, this appears to be cooking the books by data selection. However none of the allegations against Millikan appear to have involved or arisen from comments made by scientists trained in research and experimentation. David Goodstein has written in defence of Millikan and, having examined his notebooks, points out that many of the entries they contain relate to periods in which Millikan was refining his apparatus; others were simply about incomplete experiments or ones when apparatus did not function properly and a full set of data could not be collected.[18] This explanation would concur with experience in biology where, for example, a scientist working with isolated cells may find that a preparation fails to behave correctly thus meaning an experiment cannot be completed. Although some data may have been collected during an early part of the study, data from such an incomplete study might not be included in a final analysis.

What the cases of Mendel and Millikan show is that, while fraud in science is real, alive and well, its detection and management are serious matters that require serious handling. It does no good service to society in general or science in particular to have reputations destroyed and characters assassinated by unsubstantiated allegations. Sloppy or vexatious accusations fall on the same hurdle as sloppy or fraudulent science. And yet the tendency is for allegations, once made, to be repeated without a critical assessment of their validity when it suits a pitch being made as, for example, the Mendel and Millikan allegations were in *The Economist* in 2009.[19] Institutions are therefore wise to take sufficient time to investigate allegations properly and to avoid jumping to conclusions to meet news deadlines.

Fraud in Biomedical Science

Surveys suggest that scientific misconduct may be more common among medical graduates than in other fields.[2] However there is no direct evidence to confirm this and an alternative explanation could be a greater readiness on the part of this group to report it. In any event, fraud in biomedical science has certainly received great attention in the past decade. The issue is felt to be of particular importance in medicine as it may impact the lives of patients, but of course it is not unique in this respect, especially if one considers, for example, the consequences of a bridge or building being designed or built with concealed defects. What is clear is that fraud in biomedical science has the potential to harm and this may have wide-ranging consequences if it influences the treatment of many patients.

Many examples of fraud in biomedical science have been exposed in recent years. The case of South Korean Hwang Woo Suk's claim to have cloned stem cell lines from the DNA of patients using human eggs raised great hopes and expectations. The 2005 paper in *Science*,[20] which included Gerald Schatten, a stem cell scientist at the University of Pittsburgh, as senior author, offered the promise of the ability to create cultures of human tissues which could be used to repair damaged organs. It was later revealed that the study had used about six times as many eggs as claimed in the paper and that some had been obtained unethically from staff of the laboratory involved, while others had been obtained illegally from paid donors. The University of Seoul investigated the affair and announced that the authors could produce no data to support their findings. The publication had raised great hopes among patients and also expectations that South Korea was about to become a major global centre for biomedical science, the result of heavy investment in Hwang's laboratory. The disappointment was keenly felt and is likely to discourage future investment by funders and governments.

The case of fabrication uncovered in papers published by the Laboratory of Gene Transfer at the US National Institutes of Health was triggered by a careful reviewer who suspected intentional deception in a manuscript submitted for publication. The investigation that followed led to admissions by the laboratory head, Francis Collins, of fabrication and deception in several publications,[21] one of which was retracted.[22] This case raises important questions about supervision and mentoring of research students; if an external reviewer could detect deception at the Laboratory of Gene Transfer, it is difficult to envisage how careful supervision would have failed to do so. There are also questions about how much meaningful supervision one individual can provide and who should properly and fairly investigate a fraud of this kind: the laboratory involved or the institution in which it operates.

In 2005, a paper published in *The Lancet* claimed that anti-inflammatory drugs could reduce the incidence of mouth cancer. The research was based on databases of patients that included a cohort of subjects in Norway. On reading the paper, the scientists responsible for this cohort realised that the patients could not have been involved in the study without the scientists' knowledge and raised the alarm. *The Lancet* published a note of concern and the University of Oslo set up a commission to investigate the affair. The investigation concluded that data had indeed been fabricated and the paper was retracted.[23]

The Measles Mumps Rubella Affair

The most notorious, long-running and damaging example of fraud in medical science in recent years concerned the measles, mumps and rubella (MMR) vaccine in the UK. The triple vaccine was introduced in the UK in 1988. Incidence of measles increased sharply in 1994 and a vaccination campaign to promote uptake of the vaccine was launched by the Department of Health in the same year. This course of action dramatically increased the uptake of the vaccine and the incidence of measles declined thereafter.[24] Parents who were worried about possible brain damage, allegedly caused by the MMR vaccine, launched a campaign against the vaccine in 1994. In 1998, *The Lancet* published a paper by Andrew Wakefield and others suggesting a link between the MMR vaccine and autism.[25] In the same issue of the journal an editorial appeared drawing attention to the weakness of Wakefield's evidence and the dangers of confusing causality and association. It also warned of the possible tragedy that could follow if media-inspired public alarm led to parents avoiding the immunisation of their children.[26] In the event, several newspapers launched campaigns supporting Wakefield and the campaign being run by concerned parents. Uptake of the triple vaccine among children under 24 months declined from just over 88% in 1998 to under 80% by 2003.[27] It seems, however, that the use of alternate vaccines continued at a sufficient rate to avoid a further outbreak of the kind seen in 1994.[24]

Newspaper articles appeared in 2004 revealing that the Legal Aid Board had funded Wakefield's research and that some of the children involved were from families involved in litigation against the manufacturers of the MMR vaccine. This had not been declared at the time the article was published, breaching rules requiring authors to declare conflicts of interest. In the same year, most of Wakefield's co-authors retracted their interpretation that the MMR vaccine was associated with bowel and behavioural disorders. The affair was subsequently investigated by the UK's General Medical Council (GMC). The outcome of this revealed that claims made in the paper regarding ethics approval and the manner in which patients were referred were false. As a result, the entire paper was retracted by *The Lancet* in 2010.[28]

The MMR case involved several different breaches of normal ethical standards as well as authoring guidelines, and a failure by the journal editors to spot these before publication. To be fair to the editors, they did include a well-written editorial alongside the paper that cautioned about over-interpreting its findings and warned of the dangers of over-reacting to such weak evidence. In the event, this proved to be prophetic. The affair was complicated by simultaneous legal proceedings on which the work could have had a potential impact if it had proven to be correct. Furthermore, media interest in the case was intense, with some newspapers seeking to expose the work as fraudulent, while others ran campaigns in support of it and families involved in legal claims against the makers of the MMR vaccine. These competing interests may explain why the affair dragged on for so long. Wakefield's original 1998 paper was finally retracted after a lengthy enquiry by the GMC, 12 years after its initial publication. Many commentators expressed dismay that the case had taken so long to resolve and demanded more effective and rapid means to resolve such cases in the future.

Reviewing a series of case studies such as these creates a daunting picture of science riddled with dishonesty and deceit. Recent revelations of misconduct have led to understandable anger and frustration, as if it were a unique phenomenon of modern science. However it would be wrong to think of such fraud as something new; as discussed above, evidence of such misconduct extends back as far as we are able to look. The enterprise of science has dramatically increased during the past century. As rich nations have sought to become knowledge-based economies their investment in science, including both education and research, has increased greatly. This also occurred in biomedical science during the 20th century, initially to combat illness, and later for economic reasons as the demand for advanced medical products increased. There are many more scientists now and some of them will go astray, so that even if the percentage of miscreants remains unchanged the total number will still have increased. The communications revolution has allowed much greater access to the scientific literature, affording more and easier opportunities for plagiarism. Software for its detection has also become available and implementation of it by journals for routine checking of submitted manuscripts should help to drive such practices out. But humans are adaptable and who knows when we may see the introduction of language compilers to 're-write' previously published material, so that the problem shifts from plagiarism of words to one of thoughts and ideas. It seems to me that expectations that science misconduct can be 'stamped out' are not realistic; it may be wiser to accept that it has always been and will remain with us and develop better systems to improve its detection and prevention. Better understanding of how fraud is motivated and perpetrated would assist in prevention through education and removing the conditions that increase its likelihood. Clearly suspected science misconduct needs to be investigated carefully; self-appointed vigilantes have no place in this. As discussed above, false allegations do arise and can lead to erroneous judgments; false claims of scientific fraud and the consequent destruction of reputations and characters may be just as serious as fraud itself.

Detection and Prevention of Research Fraud

The scientific community is accustomed to the idea that some results that are initially thought to be correct are eventually shown to be wrong. Most of these corrections occur early, but some may elude us for a long time. For example, in the 20th century we saw Newton's law of gravity overturned, but the occasion was one of celebration for the new insights that theoretical physics had achieved and Newton's achievement was held in no less regard. By the same token, scientists should include a degree of scepticism in their thinking, so that if a new concept or idea is proposed, it is not accepted without confirmation. The occasional cheat would not seriously impair this method unless the error is repeated. That may occur, as in the N-ray case, but such an occurrence is extremely rare. In other words, misconduct has not been a serious threat to the achievements of science and therefore may have been condoned to a degree, seen as part of the inevitable disappointing failures along the way. For example, the Piltdown Man affair is often described as a hoax as though it were a clever trick rather than straightforward fraud. Perhaps there is even a small element of admiration for the way the perpetrators were able to fool so many for so long by applying expert knowledge to make the bone fragments appear to fit the theory proposed?

We do not have any measurements to allow an accurate assessment of whether the problem is more or less prevalent now than in former times, however I find it hard to believe that people today are any more or less corrupt than our forebears. It seems likely that the incidence of fraud in science appears to be greater today because of its greater role in the modern world and because more people are involved in science than formerly. Finally, if science was truly corrupt and riddled with dishonesty, it is inconceivable that the advances made in the past century could have been possible. What is clear however is that formal systems for the detection and prevention of fraud in science are inadequate and recent well-publicised cases have led to demands for action. The length of the GMC enquiry into the MMR affair was seen by some as the medical establishment dragging its heels. Others complain that academic institutions have been slow to investigate errant researchers who have been successful in attracting research grants. What then can be done? What has been done and what should be done?

Reforming the Publication Process

In most cases of misconduct, it has been the publication process that has initiated the suspicions which led to exposure, whether at the review stage or later when papers are read by the wider research community. This has been a great strength of science, but late detection, that is, after publication, is extremely wasteful of resources and has the potential to mislead other workers. Journal editors have been stung by the failure of their review procedures to identify cases in order to prevent publication and have been most active in pursuing reform, initially by establishing a code of publication ethics.

Committee on Publication Ethics (COPE)

In 1998 journal editors from around the world formed the Committee on Publication Ethics (COPE) and produced guidelines for good publication practice, which in 2011 were refined and published as codes of conduct for editors[29] and publishers.[30] These set out responsibilities for editors (Box 4.3) and include being accountable for everything published in their journal. Editors should maintain ethical relations with readers, authors, reviewers and journal owners, and ensure that submitted manuscripts are reviewed in an unbiased manner and that reviewers are informed of this responsibility and of the need to maintain confidentiality. Editors should also ensure that the research they publish complies with accepted ethical standards and that if fraud is suspected, it is investigated. These are important reforms which should help to establish new standards of working.

Box 4.3

Code of Conduct for Journal Editors

- Being accountable for everything published
- Maintaining ethical relations with journal owners, readers, authors and reviewers
- Ensuring peer review is fair, unbiased and timely
- Ensuring submitted manuscripts are kept confidential
- Encouraging ethical research
- Ensuring suspected fraud is investigated

(Committee of Publication Ethics)

Having made these changes, journal editors and other academics called for action to be taken beyond the remit of the publication process, with an emphasis on establishing a national framework to tackle the problem.

Regulating Research

The United States has already acted on the problem of research misconduct. The Office of Research Integrity (ORI) in the US was formed in 1992 by the consolidation of the Office of Scientific Integrity (OSI) and the Office of Scientific Integrity Review (OSIR), which had been set up to deal with research misconduct. In 1992 the Department of Health and Human Services set up a system for hearing cases of research misconduct before a Research Integrity Adjudications Panel. In 1999 the role of the ORI was redefined[31] (Box 4.4) to reflect the function of research institutions to investigate allegations of research misconduct. The ORI's role, mission and structure were refocused on preventing research misconduct and promoting research integrity through oversight, education and review

---

Box 4.4

The Role of the US Office of Research Integrity

- To detect, investigate and prevent research misconduct
- To review and monitor research misconduct investigations
- To assist in the presentation of cases before the Appeals Board of the Department of Health and Human Services
- To assist institutions in responding to allegations of research misconduct
- To promote education about the responsible conduct of research, to prevent research misconduct and to improve the handling of research misconduct
- To build a knowledge base in research misconduct in order to promote detection and prevention
- To assist protection of whistleblowers and respond to Freedom of Information requests

of institutional investigations.[32] The ORI has continued to develop its educational role, providing guidance for institutions, researchers and students in developing programmes to promote the responsible conduct of research.

The UK Research Integrity Office (UKRIO) was launched in 2006 and sees its role as providing independent support to research organisations in investigating misconduct (Box 4.5). UKRIO offers advice only and has no mandatory powers. It does not directly investigate misconduct, but has published a detailed procedure for investigating allegations for use by institutions and employers, and maintains a panel of advisors to assist on request. UKRIO also offers educational support relating to research ethics, but it still has some way to go in developing its educational outreach.

Research governance has increased internationally with systems either established or being developed in most countries. In China, research output has grown rapidly in recent years and is now second only to the US in the number of papers published. However the pace of growth has simply outstripped China's systems of governance and a large number of papers based on falsified data were published in 2006 and 2007,[33] prompting the government to introduce reforms.

Box 4.5

UK Research Integrity Office

Aims:

- To retain the public's trust
- To further enhance the country's international reputation
- To secure the best return on public funds
- To help ensure the safety and wellbeing of research participants and patients

Operational practice:

- Reflects best research practice
- Shares experience
- Offers advice only
- Has no mandatory powers

The publication of new cases of science misconduct inevitably leads to repeated demands for more action to combat such behaviour. However it is clear that governments and academic institutions have responded. Medical scientists who transgress face potential harsh punishment through national regulatory systems. Many commentators, particularly in the general media, feel that the time taken to bring cases to resolution is far too long, usually referring to the MMR affair as an example.[34] But considering how complex such cases can be, as illustrated by the case histories above, a rapid response may not be possible or desirable. False allegations are just as bad as science fraud and will bring any system of regulation into discredit. Careful, deliberate, fair and unbiased mechanisms are essential to ensure best practice, and it will inevitably take time to investigate allegations. Regulators such as the ORI in the US and UKRIO both recognise the need for timely action on such matters and offer assistance to institutions during investigations. Furthermore, the MMR case had its roots in a publication in 1998, before the present regulatory systems were devised and put in place. Governments, research funders, publishers and research institutions have all learned to their cost that inaction is not an option in handling misconduct and we can expect to see more exposures in the medium term as the new regulatory measures bed in.

Prevention of Fraud

In the longer term, prevention of misconduct will be crucial. In the US this appears to have been recognised early on as efforts were refocused on education as well as providing assistance to institutions in investigating cases. Ensuring that graduate students understand the importance of research integrity for their own work as well as for the future of science should be in every student's curriculum. They should also be made aware of the systems in place to detect misconduct and the consequences of straying. Supervision and mentoring are also key aspects. Research students working alone with little supervision and under intense pressure to get results is a recipe for disaster. It is also evident that many cases of fraud involve multiple authors, indicating problems in the department or institution in which it occurred. It will be important that investigations of misconduct are extended to consider these aspects also so that remedial action can be taken to prevent similar events occurring in future.

The debate about how research misconduct is investigated will continue for some time. A new wave of concern about the subject emerged in 2011 and early 2012 when the *BMJ* mounted a campaign, with the aid of investigative journalists, that resulted in the editor writing to the UK parliament requesting a judicial review of the issue.[35-39] The approach taken underscores the difficulties in tackling the matter. There is no doubt that the subject of medical fraud is of wide interest and makes for attention-grabbing headlines, but the *BMJ*'s approach appeared to be based on conversations with a few individuals,[35] lacked objective data and looked worryingly like media journalism geared to attracting readers rather than advancing an objective analysis.[36] It was not really surprising that the UKRIO later complained about inaccurate statements concerning its work.[40] The *BMJ* series was followed by calls for a new UK forensic system for investigating and policing research, the conclusion having been reached that existing mechanisms are not up to the job.[39] This was argued because of two well-known and complex cases, the MMR scandal and false accusations against paediatricians at Stoke on Trent.[41] Both of these involved intense media and political lobbying alongside determined litigation, which resulted in protracted and controversial investigations. While no one can be happy about the two cases cited, they are hardly a reasonable basis on which to suggest that existing mechanisms are incapable of adapting and that they should be side-stepped and replaced by a whole new bureaucratic structure endowed with new powers to direct and regulate research. It seems to me that in the MMR case, a new bureaucracy would not have fared much better in reaching a judgement, given its complexity and the wider media, legal and political interests involved. Furthermore the intensity of the campaign and media interest surrounding the paediatricians at Stoke on Trent reflects a malaise that would not have been responsive to calm discourse irrespective of the bureaucracy which conducted it. Legal action to challenge unfair reporting[42] and unfair trials[43] is needed to ensure that the necessary reforms are made.

The problem with this campaign is that it looks and feels more like lobbying based on generating public outrage rather than providing a balanced commentary. This weakens what should be a strong objective and respected voice. Demands for rapid detection and punishment of fraud are easy to make, but fall short of what is needed. Solutions need to take a much more comprehensive approach. Science misconduct damages society, including patients and science itself. Solutions should have the protection of all of these elements as their primary objective, which requires an understanding of the extent of the harm caused by misconduct and how science works. It is only in this way that the problem can be properly managed to include prevention, detection and correction.

To appear to resist demands for action on an issue such as science fraud risks accusations of heel dragging, or worse. However it is not difficult to find examples of well-intentioned but poorly thought-out measures which have resulted in inappropriate regulations that have themselves caused serious harm to medical science.

Inappropriate Regulation

It is clearly important that efforts to improve the regulation of medical science do not end up damaging it. This could happen if systems are introduced which fail to recognise the role and value of science and result in over-burdensome and inappropriate regulation. The primary purpose of regulation should be to protect the public and also science itself from harm. The European Union Clinical Trials Directive is a good example of inappropriate regulation. This directive was introduced in 2001 in an attempt to establish uniformity of clinical trials in the EU. It proved so complex and burdensome that it has seriously damaged clinical research in the UK. The Academy of Medical Sciences reported that clinical trials in the UK as a percentage of the global effort fell from 6% in 2000 to 2% by 2005, mainly due to difficulties with regulatory requirements arising from the EU Directive.[44,45] The Academy's reports and the government's response[45] finally recognised this and addressed the situation by creating a new Health Research Regulatory Agency to streamline regulation, including moderating the implementation of the Clinical Trials Directive. These recommendations came 11 years after the introduction of the Clinical Trials Directive and only after serious harm had already been done to clinical research in the UK. Such an example shows how badly-designed regulation, however well-intended, can cause serious harm. This has important implications for any regulator working in the field of science. There needs to be a commitment to act so as to protect science as well as the public; scientists who are currently active need to be involved in designing and implementing its functions to ensure that the way science works at the bench level is understood and can be protected.

Summary and Conclusions

Fraud in science wastes resources, misleads honest scientists in their work and undermines the integrity of the entire enterprise of scientific research. Recent examples in biomedical science have received significant publicity and caused widespread alarm.

Surveys of scientists across a range of specialties suggest a prevalence of about 2–4% of fraud within the community, with a somewhat higher rate among medical scientists. However these are limited to self-reports; objective data is not available. Reliable evidence of changes over time is also not available; the rate of self-admission appears to have declined, but it is unclear whether this is real or due to a change in reporting behaviour.

Examples of documented science fraud reveal a long-standing history of the practice and an extremely wide variety of methods, including forgery, falsifying data and physical evidence, conflicts of interest and misconduct during the publication process. There are also examples of scientists being falsely accused of misconduct due to incompetence on the part of some investigators.

Cases of science misconduct uncovered in the past two decades have led to the development of systems to improve its detection and investigation in many countries. These have been most effectively established in the US, which is the only country with a significant commitment to the prevention of science fraud through education and deterrents.

It is also recognised that poor or inappropriate regulation can damage science. The EU Clinical Trials Directive is widely believed to have seriously damaged medical science and it has taken over a decade to reform it. Further reform of science regulation is needed, in particular better understanding of the motivation of fraud and how it is perpetrated. It will also be important to monitor these systems to ensure that they make an effective contribution not only in detecting and investigating wrongdoing, but also in preventing it.

References

1. Wilkie, T., Sources in science: who can we trust? *The Lancet*, 1996; 347, 13008–13011.
2. Fanelli, D., How many scientists fabricate and falsify research? A systematic review and meta-analysis of survey data. *PloS One*, 2009; 4, e5738.
3. Ryan, K.J., Research misconduct in clinical research: the American experience and response. *Acta Oncologica*, 1999; 38, 93–97.
4. Duke, D., Ptolemy's treatment of the outer planets. *Arch. Hist. Exact Sci.*, 2005; 59, 169–187.
5. Alder, K., History's great forger: science, fiction, and fraud along the Seine. *Critical Inquiry*, 2004; 30, 702–716.
6. Smith Woodward, A. and Dawson, C., Description of the human skull and mammalian mandible and the associated remains. [A. S. W.] *Quarterly Journal of the Geological Society*, 1913; 69, 124–144.
7. Discovery of a new type of fossil man. *BMJ*, 1912; 2(2712), 1719–1720.
8. The Piltdown man discovery: unveiling of a monolith memorial. *Nature*, 1938; 142, 196–197.
9. Weinenreich, F., Skull of *Sinanthropus pekinensis*: A comparative study on a primitive hominid. *Palaeontologia Simica*, 1943; 10, 1–298.
10. Weiner, J.S., Oakley, K.P. and Le Gros Clark, W.R., The solution of the Piltdown problem. *Bulletin of the British Museum of Natural History, Geology*, 1953; 2, 139–146.
11. McLachlan, J.C., Integrative medicine and the point of credulity. *BMJ*, 2010; 341, 1312–1322.
12. Wood, R.W., The N-rays. *Nature*, 1904; 70, 530–531.
13. Lorenz, E., Search for mitogenetic radiation by means of the photoelectric method. *J. Gen. Physiol.*, 1934; 17, 843–862.
14. Fleischmann, M. and Pons, S., Electrochemically induced nuclear fusion of deuterium. *J. Electroanal. Chem.*, 1989; 261, 301–308.
15. Fisher, R.A., Has Mendel's work been rediscovered? *Annals of Science*, 1936; 1, 115–136.
16. Hartl, D.L. and Fairbanks, D.J., Mud sticks: on the alleged falsification of Mendel's data. *Genetics*, 2007; 175, 975–979.
17. Holton, G., Subelectrons, presuppositions, and the Millikan-Ehrenhaft dispute. *Historical Studies in the Physical Sciences*, 1978; 9, 161–224.

18. Goodstein, D., In defense of Robert Andrews Millikan. *Engineering and Science*, 2000; 4, 31–38.
19. Fraud in science: Liar! Liar!, *The Economist*, 3 June 2009.
20. Hwang, W.S., Patient-specific embryonic stem cells derived from human SCNT blastocysts. *Science*, 2005; 308, 1777–1783.
21. Greenberg, D.S., US genome chief withdraws five papers over fraud. *The Lancet*, 1996; 348, 1303.
22. Hajra, A., Liu, P.P., Speck, N.A. and Collins, F.S., Overexpression of core-binding factor alpha (CBF alpha) reverses cellular transformation by the CBF beta-smooth muscle myosin heavy chain chimeric oncoprotein. *Mol. Cell Biol.*, 1995; 15, 4980–4989.
23. Horton, R., Retraction-non-steroidal anti-inflammatory drugs and the risk of oral cancer: a nested case-control study. *The Lancet*, 2006; 367, 382.
24. Jick, H. and Hagberg, K.W., Measles in the United Kingdom 1990–2008 and the effectiveness of measles vaccines. *Vaccine*, 2010; 28, 4588–4592.
25. Wakefield, A.J., Ileal-lymphoid-nodular hyperplasia, non-specific colitis, and pervasive developmental disorder in children. *The Lancet*, 1998; 351, 637–641. Retracted 2010; 375, 445.
26. Chen, R.T. and DeStefano, F., Vaccine adverse events: causal or coincidental. *The Lancet*, 1998; 351, 611–612.
27. Burgess, D.C., Burgess, M.A. and Leask, J., The MMR vaccination and autism controversy in the United Kingdom 1998–2005: inevitable community outrage or a failure of risk communication? *Vaccine*, 2006; 24, 3921–3928.
28. Retraction–Ileal-lymphoid-nodular hyperplasia, non-specific colitis, and pervasive developmental disorder in children. *The Lancet*, 2010; 375, 445.
29. Committee on Publication Ethics, Code of conduct and best practice guidelines for journal editors. http://www.publicationethics.org/files/Code_of_conduct_for_journal_editors_Mar11.pdf. Accessed 5 July 2012.
30. Committee on Publication Ethics, Code of conduct for journal publishers. http://www.publicationethics.org/files/Code%20of%20conduct%20for%20publishers%20logo_0.pdf. Accessed 5 July 2012.
31. Office of Research Integrity. http://ori.hhs.gov/about/. Accessed 5 July 2012.
32. Office of Research Integrity. http://ori.hhs.gov/. Accessed 5 July 2012.
33. Scientific fraud: action needed in China. *The Lancet*, 2010; 375, 94.
34. Godlee, F., Institutional research misconduct. *BMJ*, 2011; 343, 971–972.

35. Godlee, F., Research misconduct is widespread and harms patients. *BMJ*, 2012; 344, e14.

36. Dyer, C., Calling time on research's Wild West. *BMJ*, 2011; 343, d4017.

37. Tavare, A., Managing research misconduct: is anyone getting it right? *BMJ*, 2011; 343, d8212.

38. Godlee, F. and Wager, E., Research misconduct in the UK. *BMJ*, 2012; 344, d8357.

39. Chalmers, I. and Haines A., Skilled forensic capacity is needed. *BMJ*, 2011; 343, d3977.

40. Parry, J., Reported inaccuracies about the UK Research Integrity Office. *BMJ*, 2012; 344, e547.

41. Hey, E. and Chalmers, I., Mis-investigating alleged research misconduct can cause widespread, unpredictable damage. *J. R. Soc. Med.*, 2010, 103, 133–137.

42. Parker, G., Consultant wins £625,000 damages from newspaper. *Financial Times*, 24 February 1996.

43. Dyer, C., Southall plans to sue the GMC for delays and unfair trial. *BMJ*, 2012; 344, e954.

44. Academy of Medical Sciences, Reaping the rewards: a vision for UK medical science. January 2010. http://www.acmedsci.ac.uk/p99puid172.html. Accessed 5 July 2012.

45. Academy of Medical Sciences, A new pathway for regulation and governance of health research. January 2011. http://www.acmedsci.ac.uk/index.php?pid=47&prid=88. Accessed 5 July 2012.

5

The Decline of Biomedical Science Despite Unprecedented Technological Advances: A 21st Century Paradox

In the modern world, science and technology play a major part in almost every aspect of our lives. For example, advances in methods of communication have had a major impact on the way we live and relate to each other, and how we are governed. Scientific knowledge is regarded as key to our economic success and has been the bedrock of the improvements in health and longevity that we currently enjoy. Science now operates in an ever-widening global arena in which international collaborative networks play an increasing role. The Royal Society in the UK estimates that about 7 million researchers around the world will spend over US$1,000 billion in 2011, a 45% increase since 2002.[1] The US, Japan and Europe still dominate the scientific landscape, but China has risen rapidly in recent years and India, Brazil, Southeast Asia and the Middle East are also emerging as important new centres. Recognition of the importance of science for economic development and for tackling global challenges such as health inequality, food production and climate change has been a stimulus for establishing international collaborative networks. Thus, science is flourishing; its role in shaping the future is secure with an expanding global footprint.

Many indicators of biomedical science performance also suggest a successful enterprise. Unprecedented advances were made during the 20th century in all fields of medicine, including diagnostic methods and new treatments, which have greatly improved our health and prolonged our lives. Analysis of the number of biomedical science publications indicates a continuing high level of productivity. Discoveries, such as stem cells with the potential to be transformed into any cell type to assist repair of organ damage, have captured the public imagination and raised expectations of future advances. Successes in genetics, such as the Human Genome Project, offer the possibility to understand at the most fundamental level how our bodies function as well as opportunities to intervene when things go wrong. The Academy of Medical Sciences, the Medical Research Council (MRC) and the Wellcome Trust commissioned a joint study of the economic benefits that flowed from investment in cardiovascular and mental health research in the UK between 1975 and 1992. This showed a contribution to the GDP and health gains (based on a nominal value of increased survival and quality of life) equivalent to around 39% and 30% respectively per year in perpetuity.[2] By all of these appearances therefore biomedical science is doing well. However if we look more closely it becomes clear that all is not well.

Biomedical Science in Decline

As I write, the UK Royal College of Surgeons has published a report claiming that surgical research is failing in the UK.[3] Funding of surgical research by the MRC and National Institute of Health Research in 2008/9 was less than 2% of their combined budget, and yet surgery provides a major plank of modern medical care. How can such a discrepancy exist? The stock reply from funders, 'we wish there were more applications for funds from surgeons', hardly reflects a serious engagement with what lies behind the problem. Psychiatrists and cardiologists are concerned that research into new drugs in their specialties is under threat[4,5] as the industry withdraws from these areas.

The Academy of Medical Sciences has also recognised a major gap between discoveries in basic science and putting them into practice to help patients.[6] Their report attributed the problem to a failure of clinicians to keep up with developments in molecular biology and genetics, and concluded that basic science has eclipsed clinical science. This however seems an over-simplification of the problem. It misses the critical point that success in biomedical science is dependent on clinicians and biologists working in close collaboration rather than on parallel tracks and risks diverting attention from a deeper enquiry into what lies behind the failure to deliver. Termed the 'translation gap', much has been written about fixing it and the need for 'translational research', but as yet there is little evidence of tangible improvement.

The pharmaceutical industry, which was so successful in the second half of the 20th century, is now struggling with the development of new drugs and is showing reduced research productivity. The picture of decline in the past two decades is most frequently illustrated with the fall in the number of new drugs approved, down from 53 in 1996 to 17 in 2007, but these figures are misleading since 1996 was an exceptional year. In fact, figures for new drug approvals appear stable, or slightly improved, if examined in the context of the past five decades.[7] What is unmistakable is the dramatic and continuing decline in research productivity when expressed relative to investment. While R&D spending by big pharma has increased from less than $1 billion per year in 1970 to an estimated $80 billion today, the number of new drug approvals per year has only increased slightly, while the cost of bringing a new drug to market has increased by sixfold since 1979 and is currently at around $1 billion.[7] That science and investment in science have reached peaks unheard of in history at a time when biomedical science is struggling is surely a paradox unique to the 21st century, and one that must be of wide interest to governments and policy makers. And yet explanations appear elusive. Everywhere we look we find new initiatives to 'bridge the gap', to strengthen 'translational research', to keep science 'in step with society' with little evidence of a recovery.

In this chapter, I will examine some of the reasons for this failure and why a redirection of priorities is needed. It is clear that biomedical science both enjoyed remarkable support and achieved great success until recently. The past three decades has been a period of striking change in the environment in which biomedical science operates, and it seems appropriate to begin by asking whether all of these changes have been beneficial, or whether some, however well-intentioned, have been harmful.

Clinical Research Sidelined in Health Reforms

The past three decades have seen unprecedented and repeated reforms of health care in many developed countries. The need to reduce health care costs due to increased demand and higher than average inflation has pressed governments to find new efficiencies. Platoons of economists, management advisors and think tanks have encouraged waves of reforms, which continue today. It must be said that increases in patient throughput and reduced waiting times have been achieved during this period, although it is still unclear whether and to what extent reforms contributed to this, since funding also increased substantially during the same period. However fundamental and radical changes in leadership, management style and set priorities[8] have degraded the environment which previously supported medical science and the vital links between clinicians and basic research. The decline of research in clinical settings is increasingly recognised as one of the major factors responsible for the failures of biomedical science in recent years. In other words, the reason so little funding goes to support surgical research[3] is not because funders are unwilling to support it, but rather because surgeons work in an environment which is hostile to medical science; they find it increasingly difficult to undertake the preliminary work and grant writing that is needed for a successful funding application. For the same reasons, fewer clinical scientists are able to contribute to the committee work involved in grant review and selection, which further marginalises their involvement.

In the UK, teaching and research were considered essential and intrinsic components of the NHS in that they provided for the training of future health workers and facilitated advances in biomedical science that would benefit patients. In the US and other countries, health care payments included a component that also provided for this. Recent health reforms have introduced target-driven management systems in which professional autonomy, accountability and self-motivation are replaced by imposed goals assessed by measured outputs. Targets chosen for monitoring are limited and reflect current economic and political priorities. But, as discussed in Chapter 2, the benefits of medical science may be unpredictable or not apparent for considerable periods. Consequently, science will always perform poorly in attempts at short-term measurement. Indeed it would be nonsense to compare, for example, reducing a waiting list with scientific output over a period. The result has been that medical science has been marginalised among health priorities. The damage done to academic medicine by regimes of over-administration[8] and targets focused on short-term deliverables[9] is now recognised. Participation by clinicians in medical science has been sidelined because they are coerced to work to targets[10] that take little account of their role in biomedical science. Scientific research is replaced by audits, performance measurements, health economics and re-analysis of previously published work. More worryingly, discussions about the education of future doctors often fail even to mention the words 'science' or 'research'.[11,12] Calls for a stronger representation of science at a senior level in health care planning and the need for clinical research to be enshrined in health strategy[13] are growing louder. But this would require a change in the culture that has overseen, and been partly responsible for, the recent decline, and there is little sign that this is happening yet. What is now becoming clear is that the biomedical science industry is in serious difficulty,[14] but there are a few signs that the decline in medical science which is at the heart of this is understood.

Fear and Trust

It is a paradox of the late 20th century that as the benefits of medical science increased, fear of the risks associated with medical care also increased. Thus, although we live much longer and have far better health outcomes following treatment, we are more concerned about the risks involved. This also applies to research into finding new treatments. Disasters such as those associated with thalidomide are genuine reasons why we should be seriously concerned about the risks posed by new treatments and why we should insist on measures to prevent anything similar happening again. However our fears seem to extend into a more generalised concern about medical care and in ways that are not apparent in other areas of our lives, even in those involving activities that carry even greater risks. For example, the UK had 1,900 deaths and 204,350 reported casualties on the roads in the year to September 2011.[15] We can rightly take some comfort from the fact that these figures compare favourably to those of many other developed countries, but they nevertheless represent a tremendous loss of life and most of those affected will previously have enjoyed good health. Calls for efforts to achieve greater safety are routinely met by a chorus of objections for a variety of reasons. In addition, deaths and ill health due to tobacco and alcohol use and to being overweight are now or soon will be major global epidemics, and again calls for action are regularly blunted by successful objections. The point here is that we are selective about the issues we perceive as being threats to our health and we are inconsistent in how we respond to them.

In reality, there are unavoidable risks associated with all medical treatments; by their nature all medicines interfere with the normal function of the body in some way and any such intervention cannot be undertaken without some risk. In addition, people who receive treatment are already in less than optimal health and many will be very poorly. Medical research, whether it involves healthy subjects or unwell patients, inevitably carries some level of risk to its participants' health. Consequently, there must be some reasonable benefit for the individual and to society to justify these risks. Therefore any medical research performed on live patients needs to be undertaken according to ethical rules and guidelines agreed by society so that patients are able to have trust and confidence that the work they are subject to will be carried out safely. Another consequence of increasing public concern and fear about medical care is loss of trust. As discussed in Chapter 3, although individual doctors and scientists continue to enjoy high levels of public confidence, science that is seen as being undertaken by and for the benefit of organisations, whether public or commercial, is often viewed with suspicion, as exemplified by concerns about genetically modified food and energy production. Drug development by the pharmaceutical industry also falls into this category.

Mistrust in Big Pharma

There is wide agreement that public trust in the pharmaceutical industry is low,[16,17] a situation that can only be described as a catastrophe for biomedical science. It is an irony that a system which has given us so many life-saving drugs in recent decades should now be held in such low regard. The history of medicine will remember the second half of the 20th century as outstanding for the introduction of new treatments. In my own specialty we have had new and more effective drugs to treat high blood pressure, heart failure, rhythm disturbances and high cholesterol, as well as advances in surgery, angioplasty and stents — all developments that have undoubtedly contributed greatly to reduced mortality from cardiovascular disease. The same can be said for most other branches of medicine. Attributing credit for this must recognise work done in academia and by clinicians; however a substantial part of the credit also rests with the pharmaceutical industry. How could a system which has produced so much benefit come to be held in such low esteem today? On one level, the answers are simple. New drugs have become extremely expensive as companies strive to recoup their ballooning development costs, so much so that governments struggle to meet them and have responded by building structures to restrict the use of new treatments based on measures of their cost effectiveness. The National Institute for Clinical Excellence in the UK is one of the foremost of these, and similar systems are being developed in other countries. The high cost of many drugs puts them beyond the reach of many developing countries and, as discussed in Chapter 3, has inspired the formation of global campaigns to drive down costs and to pressure governments into providing assistance. However, even in the richest countries citizens who lack health insurance can find the cost of medicines financially crippling.[18] When we add to this the greatly increased expectations about our health[19] and a growing sense that good health and access to health care is a human right,[20] these costs of medicines and the industry that makes them are increasingly perceived as a barriers to health and wellbeing. The result is that big pharma, rather than being seen as an exceptionally successful contributor to the public good, is often regarded as hostile to our best interests and entitlement. It is not my intention here to argue that our current expectations about health are reasonable or otherwise, or to make the case that access to health care is a human right, but rather to explain why the public view of the pharmaceutical industry has come to be so negative.

Industry Failures

It is also true that the pharmaceutical industry has failed to help itself. We have regular allegations of commercial malpractice such as off-label marketing (marketing for conditions not included in the approved list of indications),[21] blocking by dubious means other companies from producing cheaper generic copies of drugs when patents expire,[22] concealing information about adverse effects of drugs[23] and suing scientists over views that run contrary to commercial interests.[24] There can be no doubt that many in the pharmaceutical industry are genuinely motivated by a desire to find new treatments to improve health and must surely be dismayed by these events. However the frequency with which cases of commercial malpractice arise suggests that some in the industry must regard them as legitimate, if aggressive, practices in a competitive commercial world. But such a position loses sight of the fact that big pharma also operates in a field constrained by codes of ethics that have evolved over many centuries. Operating simply on a 'commercial perspective' or on the 'business needs' of the company is not appropriate and has caused immense harm. Huge fines handed down to Pfizer and GlaxoSmithKline[21,25] attest to the seriousness of commercial malpractice, but they do not prevent recidivism. The consequences of malpractice go far beyond any commercial costs to the companies concerned; they damage the entire enterprise of biomedical science. Involvement of paid clinicians and scientists in dubious practices, such as having their names used (whether with or without their knowledge) as authors of ghost written articles containing inaccurate information, threatens the whole scientific publication process.[26] More seriously, it undermines trust in biomedical science and the pharmaceutical industry in particular. Drug development needs close collaboration between clinical science and industry and it is generally agreed that collaboration will produce better drugs, but this collaboration is being threatened by fears that the industry is using its wealth to corrupt clinicians for marketing purposes and, in turn, by calls for the separation of clinicians and the industry.[27]

Mistrust and Regulation

A natural consequence of lack of trust is fear of unknown or hidden dangers. That in turn engenders concern and the need for caution and control. Regulation and sanctions for failure have been a feature of medical practice since ancient times, as discussed in Chapter 1, and are a major feature of modern health care. The pharmaceutical industry is a major part of the health care system and clearly needs to be regulated. The level and intensity of that regulation has increased dramatically over the past two decades and currently the industry is perhaps the most closely scrutinised on the planet. It is in itself a paradox that a system which has undoubtedly produced such outstanding benefits for society in the past and claims to be motivated to continue to do so should be so closely monitored. Why has this happened and what are the consequences? Regulators are by nature cautious. Faced with populations that are increasingly risk averse about health, they respond by adding more and more regulation. Serious adverse events during clinical trials are rare but do occur and prompt reviews of practice, which almost inevitably lead to new regulations being added. More animal studies and bigger clinical trials are required in an effort to increase public protection and so the regulations have accumulated and become more complex. Governments find it easier to add safety requirements than to remove them. Public mistrust of the industry has been particularly important in this respect as it engenders hostility among some policy makers and regulators, and constrains those who may be disposed to reform regulation. It is, I suggest, the most serious harm to have befallen the pharmaceutical industry in our time. But as I will show, the consequences are even more damaging for patients and society.

The cost of taking a new drug to the market is now thought to be about $1 billion and some have argued that this is unsustainable.[28] The high cost of development means that new drugs need to achieve peak annual sales in the region of $300 million[29]–$500 million[28] to break even. This in turn means that drug development will only be profitable in therapeutic areas where such levels of sales can be achieved, and there is ample evidence that drug development for some diseases is being adversely impacted by this. Drug development to treat diseases in the developing world has long been inadequate[30] and, as discussed above, we have recently seen large sections of the industry withdraw from R&D in mainstream therapeutic areas where the market is considered too competitive to achieve strong returns.[4,5] These decisions may be made for sound economic reasons, but the industry does not live in an economic bubble; the decisions it makes also have wide-ranging consequences for health and biomedical science.

The result is that drugs are often inadequate or lacking to treat uncommon diseases where returns are modest and therefore unlikely to be sufficient to meet development costs. More seriously, common diseases that predominantly affect poor nations fall into this category. Academia has also been severely hit; due to its close collaboration with the industry, decisions to withdraw from major therapeutic areas influences institutions to reconfigure their research portfolios to try to capture contracts, disrupting the long-term commitments in basic research that are necessary to lay the foundations for future advances. Furthermore, clinical science has become ensnared in rules and guidelines intended to regulate commercial trials for drug registration, with crippling consequences.[34] The International Conference on Harmonisation of Technical Requirements for Registration of Pharmaceuticals for Human Use (ICH) was set up by the EU in 1990 based on a steering committee of pharmaceutical industry representatives. The ICH produced a set of guidelines known as Good Clinical Practice (GCP), which were implemented to regulate commercial drug trials in Europe, Japan and the US. The WHO introduced its own version in 1995 which was heavily based on the ICH's GCP. Over time these guidelines have been applied to all research involving humans. By their nature, drug trials follow set protocols and procedures in order to provide pre-defined information for registration; the ICH and WHO guidelines were developed with this in mind and consequently are well suited for drug trials. However clinical science is concerned with original and unforeseen questions that require specifically designed and often unique study protocols to investigate them, and have great difficulty in coping with the rigidity and inflexibility inherent in the ICH and WHO guidelines. It is now widely recognised[31-35] that the guidelines have been responsible for the near crippling of original clinical research in academia, and that sensible guidelines are urgently needed.[36,37]

Mistrust Drives Fear Drives Regulation Drives Costs

A substantial reason for the ballooning cost of drug development has been the demand for more and better evidence of safety and efficacy by regulators. While regulation is understandable in the ancient sense of *premum non nocere* — first, do no harm — it nevertheless comes at a cost, which is ultimately borne by the consumers of the drugs. Michael Rawlins has argued cogently and convincingly[28] that much of this effort is no longer cost effective; the added patient safety achieved does not justify the huge costs that have now accumulated. The number of subjects involved in clinical trials to satisfy requirements for approval has more than doubled in the past two decades.[38] Much of the screening and many of the toxicology studies done during preclinical evaluation for regulatory purposes are based on a prescribed list of research steps that have never been analysed as to their actual predictive power. Rawlins argues that a great deal of this work is based on intuitive guessing and biological plausibility rather than on factual evidence. There appears to be a growing acceptance that the present model for regulation is not working and needs to change.[27] Much has been written on the subject, yet to date there is little evidence that the issue is being tackled either effectively or convincingly. Some argue for a reconfiguration of the industry to develop more targeted therapies;[39] some economists dispute that there is any problem at all, pointing to the fact that the industry has been successful in driving up prices sufficient to meet R&D costs;[40] others suggest a new model of drug development by setting up drug discovery systems in academia as a means to develop more novel drug targets;[41] while still others call for more efficient management systems to reduce costs.[39] And of course, there are calls by the industry for regulation to be relaxed.[27] However there seems little appetite for any relaxation of regulation at present and this is unlikely to change without reform of the industry itself.

Rebuilding Trust in the Pharmaceutical Industry

Reducing the ballooning cost of drug development is urgently needed. Plans to introduce 'value-based pricing' for new drugs[42] (payment based on the health benefit a drug provides, rather than its cost of development) will prevent companies from recouping large development costs of new drugs unless they offer substantial health benefits. If the industry is to remain effective in providing medicines for all aspects of health, major changes are needed in the way it works and the environment it operates in. The key to this, in my view, is restoring trust in big pharma. The dedication of the many thousands of honest workers in the industry who have provided such stunning successes in the past deserves this, but how can such a shift in perspective be achieved?

Perhaps the industry is a victim of its own success? The financial rewards that flowed from several 'blockbuster' drugs have allowed some companies to accumulate vast wealth that has turned them into corporate giants. But success has also shifted their strategic goals towards financial and economic priorities. The need to maintain competitiveness in large and lucrative markets, to protect share value and to manage global enterprises necessarily shifts attention towards managerial and financial priorities and away from science. One CEO is reputed to have told his R&D leaders that if times get tough 'the first thing we will cut is research; we know we can always increase revenues by investing more in sales'. But this is short-term folly. It feeds the kind of aggressive marketing that has caused so much damage and further erodes the science needed to break out of the poor productivity that bedevils the industry. Companies have sought to offset their failing science in the short term by using their wealth to buy smaller competitors with more promising pipelines. A further difficulty is the secrecy that is now so pervasive due to the need to protect information property. Traditionally the 'open' (i.e., published) science which takes place in academia is relied on to expand the knowledge base needed to underpin future developments. But academic institutions are already responding to tougher commercial conditions by adopting more economic tactics themselves. Thus, patents awarded to US medical schools increased dramatically between 1976 and 2003[43] and medical schools in Europe, Japan and China are following the same path. The result is a general increase in closed research or a delay in publication to secure information property rights.

It is clear that the model of drug development we have today is not sustainable and needs to change. R&D costs are far too high; the regulatory environment is excessively harsh and inflexible; attempts to streamline the process of taking drugs to market has turned the science involved into directed technical procedures and stifled original creative science. The desperate rush to recoup the high costs involved in developing new medicines has driven marketing operations in some companies to illegal activity. Trust in the industry is at a low ebb and an even harsher regulatory and economic future with value-based pricing looms. Change is needed, change that restores the industry's capacity to develop drugs as it did so brilliantly during the 20th century.

The illegal activity and sharp marketing practice that have been so damaging must end. This will require a change in the culture that operates at the top of the industry. To date, punishments handed down in the form of fines have not been a sufficient deterrent since the potential profits are also high. It needs to be recognised that the harm done goes far beyond the financial fraud involved. It undermines trust in the industry and biomedical science in general and inhibits constructive collaboration. Fines are paid as a business expense and the companies involved are essentially unaffected, as if their actions were mere corporate misdemeanours and those involved were not individually guilty. But this only serves to bolster the idea that their activities are acceptable, and even encouraged, within the corporate culture. It seems clear to me that these are major crimes that need to attract custodial punishments for those responsible. This would send a clear message that their behaviour is straightforwardly criminal and will not be tolerated. It would be a far more effective deterrent and would help to initiate the change in culture that is needed.

Science needs to be reinvigorated within the industry. By this I mean we need a return to original creative science that has proved so successful in finding new treatments in the past. The wealth accumulated from sales of successful drugs developed during the late 20th century allowed companies to invest in large-scale screening of experimental compounds against defined targets in virtually automated laboratories. This is a typical example of the application of modern management techniques to drive efficiency and productivity. Such screening appears to be highly efficient, but is intellectually rigid and lacks creative scientific input. It has failed to adapt sufficiently to the rapid evolution of biomedical science during the past decades. The process gives comfort to managers striving for efficiency but it stifles creative thinking and original science. Changing the culture at the top of the industry must include bringing real science, as distinct from rote application of technology, back into the picture.

Governments recognise the economic value and importance of the pharmaceutical industry and are keen to attract inward investment into it. However drug development tends to be viewed with suspicion, and so the stance of regulators can best be described as unconstructive. Their goal is to prevent harm, but with little thought for the consequences that follow from the conditions they lay down. They appear oblivious to the fact that they are part of the ballooning cost of drug development; the effect of the European Union's ICH-GCP and WHO's guidelines on clinical trials are clear examples of poorly thought-out regulations spilling over onto medical science, where they have had a crippling effect. Reforming the pharmaceutical industry has to include a more constructive engagement with regulators who need to consider the economic consequences of their regulations on drug making and whether the benefits they seek are cost effective, bearing in mind that this cost will ultimately be paid by consumers.

Such a system does not exist at present and would require major readjustments to the culture that currently exists among regulators, governments and the industry. It makes sense for consumers that the price they pay for new drugs should be related to the benefit they receive as a means to control costs. However, it would be unreasonable to remove from the equation the cost of meeting regulatory requirements intended to improve safety. Incentives are needed to ensure that regulations are commensurate with the costs they introduce. This would ensure that regulations are introduced to benefit patients rather than to protect regulators from criticism in the event of unforeseen adverse events. Reducing the cost of drug development will require reforming the regulations that govern the development process. The key to this is restoring trust in the pharmaceutical industry, which in turn requires a change in its corporate culture. The goal has to be to create incentives for the industry to produce more drugs at lower cost to treat all diseases based on future needs rather than on access to a few rich markets.

Summary and Conclusions

Science continues to flourish in developed countries, and this is also increasingly true in the developing world. It plays a powerful role in shaping the modern world and meeting future challenges. Advances in biomedical science during the 20th century helped to transform health care and contributed to improved health and increased longevity. However despite continued advances in the biological sciences, efforts to bring forward new developments for the benefit of patients have been in decline during the past three decades. Discoveries in basic science have not translated into health benefits and the pharmaceutical industry has experienced a marked reduction in research productivity.

These failures can be attributed to four causes:

(1) Reorganisations in the way health care is delivered in order to improve efficiency and reduce costs, sidelining clinical science and making it harder for clinicians to engage in research. Health managers often regard new treatments and innovations as cost enhancers rather than as benefits for patients.

(2) Poorly-considered bureaucratic guidelines intended to regulate commercial drug trials that have *de facto* been applied to academic clinical research with near crippling results.

(3) Mistrust of the pharmaceutical industry which has emerged as a major issue in recent years due to aggressive marketing activities that, in some cases, have amounted to fraud, with the concealment of the adverse effects of drugs, and the use of dubious legal means to thwart competitors and to silence unfavourable criticism.

(4) The cost of developing new drugs, which has increased more than tenfold over the past 30 years. This rising cost is partly due to declining research productivity in the pharmaceutical industry. It is also partly due to regulations governing the introduction of new drugs, which have accumulated over time with no consideration of their cost effectiveness and thereby of the ballooning cost of drug development.

The result is drugs that are unaffordable to many in need and a lack of drugs for rare diseases and those that occur predominantly in poor countries. We currently have a stand-off between drug makers and governments, the latter pressing for more evidence of safety to protect patients and lower drug prices to reflect the health gains the drugs provide.

Rebuilding biomedical science is needed to reverse the gap in translating scientific discoveries into health benefits; clinicians need to be involved not only in clinical research, but also in close collaboration with biological science to ensure it has relevance to practice. Management systems need to recognise the importance of autonomy, self-motivation and creativity in driving science.

The current system for regulating drug development is not sustainable. Incentives are needed for both the industry and the regulators to reduce the costs involved. This requires a more constructive engagement between governments, regulators and the pharmaceutical industry to work towards a system that relates the health benefit of new drugs to the prices they attract on the one hand and to a more shared responsibility for safety on the other, in which regulators are obliged to consider the cost/benefit of regulations they impose.

None of this can happen without the reform of the pharmaceutical industry and in particular the corporate culture that it has evolved over recent decades. Illegal and fraudulent marketing should attract custodial punishments for those involved, as well as corporate fines. Original creative science needs to be brought back into the picture to build the long-term future. In return, we need to recognise that the pharmaceutical industry has achieved stunning successes in developing new drugs in the not-too-distant past and needs to be supported in regaining that success.

References

1. Royal Society, Knowledge, networks and nations: global scientific collaboration in the 21st century. March 2011. http://royalsociety.org/policy/reports/knowledge-networks-nations/. Accessed 5 July 2012.
2. Academy of Medical Sciences, Medical research: what's it worth? November 2008. http://www.acmedsci.ac.uk/p99puid137.html. Accessed 5 July 2012.
3. Royal College of Surgeons of England, From theory to theatre: overcoming barriers to innovation in surgery. June 2011. http://www.rcseng.ac.uk/news/failure-to-support-surgical-research-will-damage-patient-care-of-the-future-warns-rcs-report. Accessed 5 July 2012.
4. Cowen, J., Has psychopharmacology got a future? *Brit. J. Psychiatry,* 2011; 198, 133–135.
5. Sheridan, D.J. and Heusch, G., Threats to the future of cardiovascular research. *The Lancet,* 2009; 373, 875–876.
6. Academy of Medical Sciences, Strengthening clinical research. October 2003. http://www.acmedsci.ac.uk/p99puid22.html. Accessed 5 July 2012.
7. Cockburn, I.M., Is the pharmaceutical industry in a productivity crisis? in *Innovation Policy and the Economy,* Number 7. National Bureau of Economic Research and MIT Press, Cambridge, Mass., 2006. http://www.hbs.edu/units/tom/seminars/2007/docs/Cockburn%20-%20Is%20-Pharma%20in%20a%20Productivity%20Crisis%20-%20scanned.pdf. Accessed 5 July 2012.

8. King's Fund, The future of leadership and management in the NHS: no more heroes. May 2011. http://www.kingsfund.org.uk/publications/nhs_leadership. html. Accessed 5 July 2012.

9. Propper, C., Sutton, M., Whitnall, C., *et al.*, Did 'targets and terror' reduce waiting times in England for hospital care? *The B E J. Econ. Analysis & Policy*, 2008; 8(2), article 5.

10. Shapiro, J. and Rashid, S., Leadership in the NHS. *BMJ*, 2011; 342, d3375.

11. The making of a modern medic. *The Lancet*, 2011; 377, 1807.

12. Frenk, J., Chen, L., Bhutta Z.A., *et al.*, Health professionals for a new century: transforming education to strengthen health systems in an interdependent world. *The Lancet*, 2010; 376(9756), 1923–1958.

13. Kmietowicz, Z., Health bill should include duty to promote medical research. *BMJ*, 2011; 342, d3196.

14. A shot in the arm. *The Daily Telegraph*, 5 December 2011. http://www. telegraph.co.uk/comment/telegraph-view/8935837/A-shot-in-the-arm.html. Accessed 5 July 2012.

15. Department for Transport, Reported road casualties in Great Britain: quarterly provisional estimates Q3 2011. February 2012. http://www.dft.gov.uk/ statistics/releases/road-accidents-and-safety-quarterly-estimates-q3–2011/. Accessed 5 July 2012.

16. PricewaterhouseCoopers' Health Research Institute, Recapturing the vision: restoring trust in the pharmaceutical industry by translating expectations into actions. 2006. http://www.pwc.com/he_IL/il/publications/ assets/11recapturing.pdf. Accessed 5 July 2012.

17. Bunniran, S., McCaffrey, D.J., 3rd, Bentley, J.P., *et al.*, Pharmaceutical product withdrawal: attributions of blame and its impact on trust. *Res. Social Adm. Pharm.*, 2009; 3, 262–273.

18. Bach, P.B., Limits on medicare's ability to control rising spending on cancer drugs. *N. Eng. J. Med.*, 2009; 360, 626–633.

19. Hart, T.J., Expectations of health care: promoted, managed or shared. *Health Expect.*, 1998; 1, 3–13.

20. Sen, A., Why and how is health a human right? *The Lancet*, 2008; 372, 2010.

21. Harris, G., Pfizer pays $2.3 billion to settle marketing case. *The New York Times*, 2 September 2009. http://www.nytimes.com/2009/09/03/business/03health.html. Accessed 5 July 2012.

22. UK sues Servier over alleged blocking of generic substitute. *BMJ*, 2011; 342, 1330–1331.

23. Psaty, B.M. and Kronmal, R.A., Reporting mortality findings in trials rofecoxib for Alzheimer Disease or cognitive impairment. *JAMA*, 2008; 299, 1813–1817.
24. A very public breakup. *BMJ*, 2010; 340, 180–183.
25. Neville, S., GlaxoSmithKline fined $3 bn after bribing doctors to increase drugs sales. *The Guardian*, 3 July 2012. http://www.guardian.co.uk/business/2012/jul/03/glaxosmithkline-fined-bribing-doctors-pharmaceuticals. Accessed 3 July 2012.
26. DeAngelis, C.D. and Fontanarosa, P.B., Impugning the integrity of medical science. *JAMA*, 2008; 299, 1833–1835.
27. Royal College of Physicians, Innovating for health: patients, physicians, the pharmaceutical industry and the NHS. Report of a working party. February 2009. http://bookshop.rcplondon.ac.uk/details.aspx?e=270. Accessed 5 July 2012.
28. Rawlins, M.D., Cutting the cost of drug development? *Nature Rev. Drug Discovery*, 2004; 3, 360–363.
29. Grabowski, H.G. and Vernon, J.M., Returns to R&D to new introductions in the 1980s. *J. Health Econ.*, 1994; 13, 383–406.
30. Ridley, D.B. and Sánchez, A.C., Introduction of European priority review vouchers to encourage development of new medicines for neglected diseases. *The Lancet*, 2010; 376, 922–927.
31. Morice, A.H., The death of academic clinical trials. *The Lancet*, 2003; 361, 1568.
32. Hemminki, A. and Kellokumpu-Lehtinin, P.L., Harmful impact of EU clinical trials directive. *BMJ*, 2006; 332, 501–502.
33. White, N.J., Clinical trials in tropical diseases: a politically incorrect view. *Trop. Med. Int. Health*, 2006; 11, 1483–1484.
34. Europe's restrictive rules strangling clinical research. *Nat. Med.*, 2005; 11, 1260.
35. Grimes, D.A., Hubacher, D., Nanda, K., *et al.*, The Good Clinical Practice Guideline: a bronze standard for clinical research, *The Lancet*, 2005; 366, 172–174.
36. Academy of Medical Sciences, A new pathway for regulation and governance of health research. January 2011. http://www.acmedsci.ac.uk/p47prid88.html. Accessed 5 July 2012.
37. Lang, T., Cheah, P.Y. and White, N.J., Clinical research: time for sensible global guidelines. *The Lancet*, 2011; 377, 1553–1555.

38. Di Masi, J., Hansen, R.W. and Grabowski, H.G., The price of innovation: new estimates of drug development costs. *J. Health Economics*, 2003; 22, 151–185.
39. WHO, Bridging the 'know–do' gap. Meeting on Knowledge Translation in Global Health 10–12 October 2005. http://www.who.int/kms/WHO_EIP_KMS_2006_2.pdf
40. McKinnon, R., Worzel, K., Rotz, G., *et al.*, Crisis? What crisis? A fresh diagnosis of big pharma's R&D productivity crunch. Research paper from Marakon Associates, New York, 2004. http://www.marakon.com/ideas_pdf/id_041104_mckinnon.pdf. Accessed 21 October 2008.
41. Tralau-Stewart, C.J., Wyatt, C.A., Kleyn, D.E., *et al.*, Drug discovery: new models for industry–academic partnerships. *Drug Discovery Today*, 2009; 14, 95–101.
42. Department of Health, A new value-based approach to the pricing of branded medicines. December 2010. http://www.dh.gov.uk/prod_consum_dh/groups/dh_digitalassets/@dh/@en/documents/digitalasset/dh_122793.pdf. Accessed 5 July 2012.
43. Azoulay, P., Michigan, R. and Sampat, B.N., The anatomy of medical school patenting. *New Eng. J. Med.*, 2007; 357, 2049–2056.

6

Changes in Medical Professionalism in the 21st Century and Their Impact on Medical Science

The word 'professional', in former times, described the entrance to a religious order. In general usage today it refers to a person engaged in one of the learned professions; in the past this also carried an implication of social superiority to those involved in trade or handicraft. The term can also mean a person who maintains a lifelong commitment to a particular form of work, such as a professional footballer or soldier. In the context of medicine however it refers to a commitment to abide by a contract between medicine and society. Medical professionalism is based on a commitment always to act in the best interests of patients and derives from the Hippocratic tradition. This has been the ethical basis of medical practice for centuries, but for several reasons medical professionalism came under close scrutiny during the late 20th century. The obligation to put the patient's best interests ahead of all other considerations appears simple enough, but it begs the question who decides what is in the patient's best interest? In former, less egalitarian times the balance of who made decisions about care rested with doctors far more than would be acceptable today; people are now much better informed and wish to be more involved in the process; differences between social groups have declined and automatic deference to figures of authority is questioned so that some have come to view the doctor–patient relationship as patronising, condescending and in need of change.

The medical profession, particularly in the United States, is often described as having enjoyed a 'golden age' after the Second World War when doctors held a powerful social position, but from about the 1950s doctors began to experience sustained criticism for being arrogant, self-interested and exercising excessive social control. Ivan Illich was the harshest of these critics, describing medicine as a systematic attack on health. He viewed the medical profession as depriving people of the ability to manage their experience of suffering.[1] He described education in much the same way, that is, as an attack on learning.[2] His thesis contained elements that found resonance with many. For example, he stressed a way of living in which self-reliance features strongly and he criticised institutional appropriation of the means for dealing with everyday discomforts; ideas that, I suspect, few doctors would disagree with.

Illich's views were widely circulated and became influential, particularly among sociologists. Extreme aspects of his criticisms, for example, that medical alleviation of pain is bad because it deprives patients of the ability to develop what he called 'the art of suffering', were largely ignored by medical professionals, who presumably regarded it as nonsense; by the public, who preferred to receive help; and even by his supporters, who were caught up in the 'religious experience' of his style of delivery. I believe that Illich's views on medicine are often misread. In fact, he made it clear that he had no interest in health.[3] He was not on a mission to reform medicine but to change the way we live, and for this goal shock tactics were his preferred method. His targets were institutions of all kinds, however his priority was the method of delivering his message rather than the message itself. This explains why his objectives are so frequently misunderstood. In this context, his disappointment with his texts being part of the curricula of the very institutions of education he condemned is revealing. Eliot Freidson's attack on US medicine was more direct and effective. He criticised doctors for being too powerful and arrogant, and for acting against the public interest,[4] and he led the charge of a number of other, mainly sociology academics against them. The growth of managed care in the US from the 1980s added to the sense that clinical freedom and medical professionalism were under threat.

Ivan Illich appears to have been more influential in the UK than in the US and he still enjoys iconic status among some commentators[5] in a campaign against over-medicalisation, but this is cherry-picking Illich's views. He was critical of medicine as an institution and I suspect he would not have welcomed the recruitment of his work into the medical establishment in this way. Thomas McKeown[6] and Archie Cochrane[7] were key figures in the UK whose criticisms of medicine have been highly influential in many countries.[8] This is partly due to the fact that the system of health care delivery in the UK has many features in common with the systems used in other countries. McKeown argued that economic and social factors account for almost all reductions in mortality and that medical contributions were negligible. Some public health experts, mainly in the US, criticised his analysis and interpretation of mortality data, arguing that a significant contribution had been made by public health measures, while happily going along with McKeown's criticisms of clinical medicine.[9,10] Cochrane also criticised clinical medicine as wasteful and inefficient and argued for evidence-based medicine based on randomised controlled clinical trials. He wrote at a time when such trials were beginning to be widely used in clinical research and, although he had very little experience of them himself, he became something of an icon in the evidence-based medicine movement that followed.

Failure of Medical Ethics and Regulation

A number of cases of serious unethical or criminal behaviour which occurred or came to light during the late 20th century added greatly to concerns about medical ethics and professionalism. In the US, the Tuskegee study of the natural progression of syphilis conducted by the Public Health Authority between 1932 and 1972 deceived its participants about the nature of the study in which they were participating, and not only withheld treatment with penicillin after it had been discovered that it could cure syphilis, but also actively hindered patients from getting treatment elsewhere. When these actions became public knowledge in 1972, the US government set up the National Commission for the Protection of Human Subjects in Biomedical and Behavioral Research to undertake a deep review of bioethics, the results of which were published in the Belmont Report in 1979.[11]

In the UK, Harold Shipman, a GP in Hyde, Greater Manchester was convicted of murdering 15 of his patients in 2000. Following a police investigation, the number of murders ascribed to him was revised to 218, and this figure may well still be an underestimate of his activities. The Shipman Inquiry[12] which followed made several far-reaching recommendations, among them the need for substantial reform of the General Medical Council, the body which regulates doctors and is responsible for maintaining their professional standards in the UK.

The report of an enquiry published in 2001[13] into an unusually high number of perioperative deaths between 1984 and 1995 at the Bristol Royal Infirmary paediatric cardiac surgical unit identified a range of serious failures and inadequacies in the health service involving funding, individual clinicians, leadership, facilities available and the organisation of the service. The report made wide-ranging recommendations for improving (i) the care children receive, (ii) the culture in which the service operates, with particular emphasis on transparency, safety, monitoring of standards and involvement of the public, (iii) management and leadership and (iv) lifetime competency of its professionals.

During the course of taking evidence at the Bristol Royal Infirmary Inquiry, it also became clear that a great deal of knowledge had been obtained from the study of hearts retained following post mortem examinations of patients with complex forms of congenital heart disease. While the benefits of this were established, it also became clear that organs had been retained and stored without the consent of parents or relatives in many cases and that this had been the wide practice for several decades. An inquiry into the Royal Liverpool Children's Hospital,[14] where the largest collection of organs in the UK was based, led to the Tissue Act 2004, which created the Human Tissue Authority to regulate the handling of human tissues in the UK.

Health Care Budgets in Crisis

These events had a profound impact on medicine in the UK. As the millennium dawned, the profession found itself buffeted and it appeared to be uncertain about the future. Many feared that the profession had lost the trust and confidence of society and that the very concept of medical professionalism and the values it espoused were threatened. But more was to come as health services around the world began to struggle with the rising costs of health care. During the early post-war period, the treatments available were simpler, less specialised and far cheaper than they are today. In the UK, spending on the NHS was around 3.5% of GDP during the 1950s.[15] Since then spending has increased substantially. NHS expenditure increased from around £2 billion in 1971/2 to around £100 billion today, the rising expenditure

> **Upheavals in Medicine 1970–2010**
> • Changing social and political attitudes
> • Failures of medical ethics led to reform of regulation
> • Crises in funding health care led to reorganisation of health care and its management

reflecting advances in treatment, specialisation and the increased expectations of patients. The figures certainly look dramatic, although when put in the context of gross domestic product which, of course, has also increased substantially during the same period, they represent an increase from about 4.5% to 10%, which is still below the European average.[17] Nevertheless, rising costs have caused increasing alarm among economists and politicians and have led to repeated attempts to reform health care. The Community Care Act in 1990 introduced an 'internal market' within the NHS in the hope that separating service procurement from provision would increase efficiency and contain costs through competition. In the event, little was achieved in terms of cost savings and a new government extended the concept to include external private providers while continuing to fund the system from taxation. Improvements in waiting times were achieved, but these were also associated with a major increase in funding of the NHS. The challenge to contain costs remained unsolved. Despite the efforts of the previous two decades, projected increases in health spending were still estimated to double by 2030, an expense which was considered unaffordable.[16] New proposals were brought forward in 2010 for yet further reforms. This new round of reforms would shift commissioning to GPs, reduce management and introduce more private health care into the NHS. By now a degree of reform-exhaustion had set in and the new proposals met more concerted opposition from clinicians and managers.[17] As I write the government is reconsidering its proposals.

Health Care Management

Thus, medicine experienced a period of unprecedented upheaval during the decades around the new millennium. But the impact on clinicians and clinical science was felt most keenly as a result of changes in the way the service was managed. Organisation of health care delivery requires systems of management, leadership, administration and bureaucracy. During most of the 20th century, clinicians and in some instances clinical academics played leading roles in managing the service. After all, medicine and medical science had made great progress during this period and so doctors were perhaps considered to be most capable of fulfilling these management and administration roles, too. This approach relied on a system in which the doctor knew what was best for patients and was committed to act in their best interests. Clinical training was geared to encourage self-direction and motivation, to question what is practised, and to seek new and better ways to diagnose and treat illness. In other words, doctors were trained to work with a high degree of autonomy, to think independently and to do what they judged to be right. This approach applied to the way medicine was practised and also to the way the health service was managed. However management systems had developed in radically different ways in almost all other areas of work during the same period (the law would be one exception). Modern management systems had contributed to dramatic improvements in industrial efficiency during the 20th century and introduction of these into health care was seen as a vital step to improving productivity and reducing costs. The consequences for medicine and medical science were dramatic and painful.

NHS Management Pre-1990

- Clinicians played a leading role
- System based on traditional ethics
  - o Acting in patients' best interests
  - o Relying on doctors' knowledge
  - o Medical independence
  - o Self-direction and motivation

A Shift of Authority

Whereas clinicians and clinical academics had taken leading roles in managing the health service in the past, new blood with new ideas were considered necessary to drive the changes that would be needed to achieve the reforms. The medical profession had originally opposed the introduction of the NHS in the UK,[18] but in the decades since, the profession was considered by reformers to have geared the service to its own advantage and it would now oppose further reforms. As in other countries, doctors' interests were felt to be too closely linked to maintaining the status quo to engage positively with change. And so a minor revolution in health care management ensued with, as one commentator put it, 'professors being deposed by CEOs'.[19] In retrospect the speed of change was remarkable. Looking back, it seems to me that morale in the profession at the time had already been buffeted by prolonged and repeated adverse media reactions to 'scandals' and 'medical blunders'. Some doctors and nurses took on management roles; there was a minor rush into MBA courses, but the majority of the profession seemed unconvinced and withdrew into clinical practice. The result was a rapid transformation with a major recruitment of managers, but with poor engagement by clinicians who maintained a rather mute resistance to the new systems of management,[20,21] which some would later blame for hampering progress.[22] But the changes represented a real shift of authority away from clinicians, and were radical in terms of the way the service was managed.

A Change in the Culture of Health Care

The culture in which health services had operated for most of the 20th century was based on high levels of trust, self-motivation and direction, beneficence (doing what was right under the circumstances) and a high level of individual clinical independence. Emphasis on the doctor–patient relationship put the individual patient's experience at the forefront. However, management systems in other industries had evolved during the same period to deliver the greater productivity and efficiency needed by large corporations and institutions, which resulted in quite a different operating culture. These management systems would begin with a systematic study of the organisation to develop an overall strategy; individual elements of the work it did would then be examined in detail to identify key tasks and roles. These functions would then be analysed and broken down into operational steps and these steps would be coordinated

Industrial Management Systems

- An organisational strategy is defined:
    o Key priority objectives
    o Operational targets
    o Performance measurement
- The 'mission' permeates the organisation
- The most efficient pathways and operational steps are defined
- Teams created to:
    o Enhance communication
    o Encourage group commitment to the culture and mission
- Individual workers encouraged to:
    o Buy in to the mission
    o Work to the agreed strategy

to achieve optimal efficiency; finally monitoring systems would be created to assess performance. The resulting culture is one in which the organisational strategy is the key driver. This defines the overall priority objectives in a context of measurable performance. It is usually expressed as a mission statement, which is intended to permeate, direct and motivate all parts of the organisation. By defining pathways and operational steps based on highest efficiency, great simplification and higher throughput are achieved. Teams are created to enhance communication and to promote group identification with the mission. These systems have proved extremely effective in increasing industrial productivity in all developed countries and political systems. However, as discussed below, their application in the field of health care has been more problematic.

Medical Professionalism and Health Service Management

It is now widely recognised that health care reforms introduced to improve efficiency and productivity failed to engage health workers adequately.[23] This is now believed to have hindered progress[21,22] and has recently begun to receive attention.[24] There are several reasons for this disconnection between health workers and those attempting to impose reform upon them. Given the central role that clinicians had played in running services in the past, there may have been concerns that they would oppose the changes (as doctors had originally opposed the introduction of the NHS) seen as being essential to reform. Consequently, new managerial blood may have been considered strategically helpful during the early stages. However engagement may also have been limited because of the nature of the discourse in driving reforms. Advances in medicine during the 20th century have been based on evidence gathered from experimental and clinical research, with peer review as a means to ensure quality. In contrast, much of the discussion around reforms and new managerial systems was derived from experience in industry and the assumption that such measures could be applied generically to health care. Although put forward with the sometimes evangelical enthusiasm of management consultants, the reforms and management systems lacked real health care experience or evidence as to their suitability to the field. Clinicians used to dealing with evidence may have found it difficult to engage in a discourse that lacked any. Calls for evidence were met with replies based on further enthusiastic rhetoric which had a tendency to stifle progress. A similar pattern emerged in the published record, which tended to rely on policy documents based on opinion and published without peer review. For example, a recent report on leadership and management in the NHS contained 55 references, only one of which related to a peer-reviewed publication containing evidence of relevant experience[24] and, like many similar reports and policy documents concerning NHS reforms, it was published 'in-house' without the scrutiny of peer review. Then there is the question of 'conflict of interest', which is almost always ignored in such publications, but which clinicians and scientists are required to declare for almost all other publications. Often even the language itself in many policy documents does not lend itself to rational dialogue. In his Rock Carling lecture,[25] Theodore Marmor, Professor Emeritus of Public Policy and Management at Yale University, criticised the quality of discussion of management in health care. In drawing attention to the 'linguistic muddle and conceptual confusion' often encountered he cited the examples of 'managed care', used as a persuasive linguistic device to promote change. He noted that in reality such terms amount to meaningless sloganeering (as if unmanaged care were a real alternative). Similarly 'integrated care' was a popular objective for progressive managers for a while (as though opponents were keen on disintegrated care). He and others[26] have noted the 'product cycle' of policy fads in health care management, as failed policies are dropped and replaced by new models. The ease with which enthusiasms initially marketed with zealous hyperbole are later casually abandoned as the proponents move on to newer concepts and fashions is reminiscent of Lysenkoism in the 1930s Soviet Union.

Jargon and Cynicism

Many health workers may be tempted to ignore the worst examples as sloganeering jargon and take the view that it can have little effect. But, as Marmor points out,[25] at the very least they take up time and energy and, more seriously, they can mislead audiences. For example, the 'purchaser–provider interface' becomes management speak for what used to be the doctor/nurse–patient relationship. It describes the interaction in organisational terms in a way that removes the experience of all those involved and implies that providing care is like any other managed item, be it nuts and bolts or apples and pears. A central theme of a recently published report on leadership and management in the NHS[24] was the concept of 'the post-heroic model of leadership'. This would downgrade the contribution of the most experienced in favour of a model where everyone becomes a leader with 'the focus on organisational relations, connectedness, interventions into the organisation systems, changing organisation practices and processes'. Again, the relationship with patients, the element most important for the professionalism of doctors and nurses, is degraded in favour of what appears to be little more than managerial jargon.

Failures in Health Care: The Patients' Experience

There is now increasing evidence that this negation of the patients' experience in favour of organisational efficiency has had serious adverse effects on care. An Independent Inquiry conducted by Robert Francis[27] into care provided by Mid Staffordshire NHS Foundation

Trust between 2005 and 2009 described widespread failings in the standard of care provided, with an 'over reliance on figures' as one of the reasons for the Trust's failings. The Inquiry described staff as being thoroughly demoralised and identified an urgent need for management to listen to and respect their professional views. That this problem has become widespread is indicated by the Health Service Ombudsman's 2011 report to parliament.[28] This was particularly critical of the neglect of patients' experience and dignity, which it described as symptomatic of a 'gulf between the principles and values of the NHS Constitution and the felt reality of being an older person in the care of the NHS in

Charter for Medical Professionalism[32]
• Fundamental principals
o Primacy of patients' welfare
o Patients' autonomy
o Social justice
• Professional responsibilities
o Professional competence
o Honesty with patients
o Patients confidentiality
o Maintaining appropriate relationships with patients
o Improving quality of care
o Improving access to care
o Fair distribution of resources
o Commitment to scientific knowledge
o Maintaining trust by managing conflicts of interest
o Maintaining standards of the profession

England'. It attributed this to 'an attitude — both personal and institutional — which fails to recognise the humanity and individuality of the people concerned and to respond to them with sensitivity, compassion and professionalism'. Similarly, the Care Quality Commission[29] reported in 2011 that 55 out of 100 hospitals evaluated were not fully compliant with standards relating to nutrition, dignity and respect. Less significant in terms of statistics, but more telling in their direct impact, are the heart-breaking stories of patients' or relatives' experiences of indifference, neglect and even cruelty[30] that suggest not just a lack of individual responsibility, but of large-scale subversion of altruism and professionalism.

The Public View of Medical Professionalism

Some might argue that health care is just another job; that being a good doctor or nurse is like any other work with no special or particular professional character. Indeed, when looked at carefully, this appears to be a prevailing view that lies behind much of the jargon and recent managerial approach to health care.[24–26] It is not the view of the general public however, as revealed by a survey of 953 individuals about the main professional attributes of doctors. Most of the respondents identified respect for patients' autonomy and dignity as the most important attributes, together with honesty and compassion.[31]

A Charter for Medical Professionalism

Around the turn of the century, physicians from many countries working in diverse health care systems became concerned that medical professionalism was being threatened by changes in health care delivery in almost all industrialized counties, and more specifically that medicine's commitment to the patient was being challenged. Subsequently meetings among the European Federation of Internal Medicine, the American College of Physicians, the American Society of Internal Medicine and the American Board of Internal Medicine recognised the need for a renewed sense of professionalism and established a charter for medicine that would be applicable to all cultures and political systems.[32] The principals on which it is based commit doctors to the primacy of patients' welfare, patients' autonomy and the elimination of discrimination in health care. Doctors must commit to maintaining professional competence, honesty, integrity, trust and confidentiality in their relations with patients and work to improve the quality and accessibility of care. In addition, doctors must commit to maintaining and developing new scientific knowledge and to supporting the standards of the profession through internal and external scrutiny. These fundamental principles and responsibilities are regarded as definitive, despite having in some instances to contend with complex and sometimes conflicting political, legal and market forces.

Preserving Medical Professionalism in Health Care Reforms

The struggle to manage health budgets by improving efficiency and productivity continues. It is clear that their commitment to professionalism obliges physicians to support these efforts. However it is equally clear that physicians have not been fully engaged in the reform process and that a lack of involvement has hampered progress.[21,22] Some advisors have suggested that doctors' and nurses' reluctance to engage in 'quality management' results from their perceived loss of control and cited the need to replace 'individual control' with 'systems control',[14] but this appears to reflect an engineering view that management systems can be generically applied and without any consideration of medical professionalism or the exceptional nature of human experience of illness. More recent commentators acknowledge that failure to incorporate the professional values of health workers as key elements of health care management has in effect excluded those workers from a more inclusive involvement in the reform process.[23] However this view is not yet widely accepted.[24] What is clear is that many reforms have failed to achieve their objectives,[33,34] wasting valuable resources. It is also clear that undermining professionalism has contributed to recent service failures[27–29] and that the medical profession is now becoming more vocal about this issue.[19,35] Similar moves are afoot in nursing.[30]

Medical Professionalism and Biomedical Science

I have devoted a lot of space to discussing factors that impact medical professionalism here because I believe that it is inextricably linked to progress and decline in medical science. As discussed in Chapter 2, the most powerful driver of scientific inquiry is curiosity: the impulse to ask why and how things are as they are. In turn, an atmosphere in which thinking and questioning are encouraged is essential for new ideas to emerge. In addition, novel concepts that can lead to medical advances require that doctors engaged in clinical practice are educated in the sciences and are supported to work in a manner that encourages research. This is not to undervalue the contribution that biological scientists make to medical progress. However it is clinical encounters between doctors and patients, and especially those that throw up new diagnostic and therapeutic challenges, which are most important for directing medical science. This is what defines new areas of research and stimulates the curiosity needed to drive it. In other words, the patient's bedside is a vital part of the biomedical science laboratory. If this is missing science will still flourish, but it is less likely to lead to medical advances and this, I suggest, is the principle reason for the 'translation gap', the failure to translate advances in biological science into new therapies and diagnostic methods, which has developed over the past few decades.

It is not difficult to envisage how a programme that induces a 'terror of targets' related to measurable performance would stifle an atmosphere of inquiry. A management culture in which the priority is to satisfy defined systems and processes relegates the experience and intellectual engagement of the clinical encounter to a transactional detail in which measurable performance is the primary objective. Those involved are groomed to prioritise responding to the requirements of the system rather than to the patient or the challenges that arise from the clinical encounter. Furthermore, as discussed above, the introduction of new management systems into health care shifted authority towards those who manage them, and inevitably resources were also prioritised to meet the performance measures defined by them. Investing in teaching and medical science would not achieve a high level of priority among the short-term measurable performance indicators in such a system and this I suggest is the principle reason for the decline of academic medicine[36,37] and the 'translation gap' that has emerged during the past two decades.

The new charter on medical professionalism includes a commitment to scientific knowledge as a key responsibility of doctors, including keeping up to date, contributing to educating others, promoting research and creating new knowledge.[32] Failure to acknowledge these commitments in prevailing management and policy strategies[23,24] seems likely to remain a stumbling block to clinicians engaging fully in reform processes. For example, a recent report on the management of health care claimed to have consulted no fewer than 23 external organisations or individuals, but not a single academic institution or research funding organisation was listed among them.[24] The most recent Health and Social Care Bill proposing wide-ranging health care reforms in the UK was widely viewed in the clinical academic community as failing to acknowledge and support research within the health service and was heavily criticised for failing to take action to reverse the decline in medical research and the consequent damage to the economy.[38,39] Indeed there are increasing signs of concern among clinical academics at what they see as a lack of vision and progress.[40]

The Way Forward?

Given the medical profession's long history and its recently renewed commitment to professionalism, it seems unlikely that the values it embodies will disappear; indeed there are signs that clinicians may be more willing to resist threats to them.[19] On the other hand, efforts to control health care costs will have to continue as, for example, the US is estimated to be on course to spend a fifth of its GDP on health by 2020.[41] For much of the past three decades the effort has been on the introduction of industrial management systems, with the promise of more streamlined operations and greater productivity. But each new system has largely failed to deliver and has been replaced by a new system. A fundamental error in all of these approaches has been the failure to recognise the key role of the professional values of doctors and nurses. Perhaps there are signs of recognition that this has de facto excluded them from the process and that this has hindered progress.[22] Harnessing the core values of professionalism is now seen as an alternative way to achieve the reforms needed.[23] Most hospitals were traditionally led by doctors, but this changed radically with the introduction of reforms and the majority of hospitals in the US and UK are now managed by non-physicians;[42,43] of the 6,500 hospitals in the US, only 235 are run by doctors.[44] And yet the available evidence indicates that hospitals led by physicians consistently perform better on a range of quality measures.[45]

However the point here is not to argue for a physician-led health care system, but rather to recognise that reforms need to engage health workers fully in order to be successful, and that means acknowledging and respecting their professionalism and the doctor/nurse–patient relationship. This would also be the means to re-energise medical research. But there is some way to go. Accepting that medical science is a core professional value that must be supported within and by health services, that medical advances need to be seen as new and better ways to treat patients rather than as added costs which threaten budgets, and that clinical research is a vital part of the economy will not be easy for a management style that relies on systems and processes and short-term measurement performance. Medicine has had its ups and downs in the past, and no doubt will again in the future. But an enduring and constant feature of it is the need of people to see a human face when seeking help during illness, and there seems no better way to protect this basic right than by ensuring that medical professionalism is preserved, irrespective of prevailing political opinions and views. This too will be the way to reverse the decline in medical research.

Summary and Conclusions

Medical professionalism came under close scrutiny with the dawn of the 21st century. Well-publicised cases of unethical or criminal behaviour and examples of poor performance led many to question the traditional view of the profession. A crisis in health care budgets led to reorganisation and the introduction of management systems which reduced the role of clinicians in management. As one editorial expressed it, 'professors were deposed by CEOs'.[46] These changes led to a shift of authority.

The reforms that followed changed the culture in which medicine is practised; trust, accountability, autonomy and independence were reduced in favour of missions, targets, team-working and performance measurement. Many of these reforms failed to meet expectations, and this can be attributed in part to a lack of engagement with health workers. This in turn reflects a widely held view that many of the reforms threatened medical professionalism; physicians from several countries, cultures and political systems reacted by establishing a new charter of professionalism which upheld many of the traditional values of medicine as a profession.

Biomedical science depends on a culture of enquiry in which questioning and freedom to explore new avenues are encouraged. These were eroded by the new management regimes which sought to prioritise efficiency through directed, target-driven teamwork backed by performance measurement. Academic medicine was degraded and the clinician-patient interaction became disconnected from mainstream biomedical science. The result is a divergence between biological science and medicine, and a breakdown of collaboration between the two which had proved so successful during the 20th century.

The current crisis in biomedical science is now well recognised. Resolving it will depend on re-establishing medical science as a core professional value, and this in turn means respecting and preserving medical professionalism as a key element of health care delivery.

References

1. Illich, I., *Medical Nemesis*. Calder and Boyers, London, 1974.
2. Illich, I., *Deschooling Society*. Calder and Boyers, London, 1971.
3. llich, I., Pathogenesis, immunity, and the quality of public health. *Qualitative Health Research*, 1995; 5(1). http://brandon.multics.org/library/Ivan%20 Illich/against_coping.html
4. Freidson, E., *Profession of Medicine: a Study of the Sociology of Applied Knowledge*. Dodd Mead, New York, 1970.
5. Moynihan, R. and Smith, R., Too much medicine? Almost certainly. *BMJ*, 2002; 324, 859–860.
6. McKeown, T., *The Role of Medicine: Dream, Mirage or Nemesis?* Nuffield Provincial Hospitals Trust, London, 1976.
7. Cochrane, A.L., *Effectiveness and Efficiency: Random Reflections on Health Services*. Nuffield Provincial Hospitals Trust, London, 1972.
8. Alvarez-Dardet, C. and Ruiz, M.T., Thomas McKeown and Archibald Cochrane: a journey through the diffusion of their ideas. *BMJ*, 1993; 306, 1252–1255.
9. Colgrove, J., The McKeown thesis: a historical controversy and its enduring influence. *Am. J. Public Health*, 2002; 92, 725–729.
10. Szreter, S., Rethinking McKeown: the relationship between public health and social change. *Am. J. Public Health*, 2002; 92, 722–725.
11. Office of Human Subjects Research, The Belmont Report: ethical principles and guidelines for the protection of human subjects of research. April 1979. http://www.hhs.gov/ohrp/archive/documents.19790418.pdf. Accessed 5 July 2012.

12. The Shipman Inquiry, Sixth report — Shipman: the final report. January 2005. http://www.shipman-inquiry.org.uk/finalreport.asp. Accessed 5 July 2012.

13. The Bristol Royal Infirmary Inquiry, The report of the public inquiry into children's heart surgery at the Bristol Royal Infirmary 1984–1995: Learning from Bristol. July 2001. http://www.bristol-inquiry.org.uk/final_report/index.htm. Accessed 5 July 2012.

14. The Royal Liverpool Children's Inquiry, The Royal Liverpool Children's inquiry report. January 2001. http://www.rlcinquiry.org.uk/. Accessed 5 July 2012.

15. Shapiro, J., The NHS: the story so far (1948–2010). *Clin. Med.*, 2010; 10, 336–338.

16. Lansley, A., Why the health service needs surgery. *The Telegraph*, 1 June 2011. http://www.telegraph.co.uk/comment/personal-view/8551239/Why-the-health-service-needs-surgery.html. Accessed 5 July 2012.

17. Appleby, J., Can we afford the NHS in the future? *BMJ*, 2011; 343, 126–127.

18. Honigsbaum, F., *Health, Happiness and Security: the Creation of the National Health Service*. Routledge, London, 1989.

19. Horton, R., The doctor's role in advocacy. *The Lancet,* 2002; 359, 458.

20. Shekelle, P.G., Why don't physicians enthusiastically support quality improvement programmes? *Qual. Saf. Health Care*, 2002; 11, 6.

21. Morrison, P.E., Heineke. J., Why do health care practitioners resist quality management? *Qual. Prog.* 1992; 25(4), 51–55.

22. Gallop, R., Whitby, E., Buchanan, D., *et al.*, Influencing sceptical staff to become supporters of service improvement: a qualitative study of doctors' and managers' views. *Qual. Saf. Health Care*, 2004; 13(2), 108–114.

23. Shapiro, J., Rashid, S., Leadership in the NHS: professionals respond better to inclusion than coercion. *BMJ*, 2011; 342, d3375.

24. King's Fund, Future leadership and management in the NHS: no more heroes. May 2011. http://www.kingsfund.org.uk/publications/nhs_leadership.html. Accessed 5 July 2012.

25. Marmor, T., Fads in medical care policy and politics: the rhetoric and reality of managerialism. Rock Carling Lecture, November 2001. http://mba.yale.edu/faculty/pdf/marmor_rockcarling110701.pdf. Accessed 5 July 2012.

26. Huczynski, A., *Management Gurus*. Routledge, London, 2006.

27. Department of Health, Independent Inquiry into care provided by Mid Staffordshire NHS Foundation Trust January 2005 — March 2009. Chaired by Robert Francis QC. February 2010. http://www.dh.gov.uk/en/

Publicationsandstatistics/Publications/PublicationsPolicyAndGuidance/
DH_113018. Accessed 5 July 2012.

28. Parliamentary and Health Service Ombudsman, Care and compassion? Report of the Health Service Ombudsman on ten investigations into NHS care of older people. February 2011. http://www.ombudsman.org.uk/care-and-compassion/downloads. Accessed 5 July 2012.

29. Care Quality Commission, Dignity and nutrition inspection programme: national overview. October 2011. http://www.cqc.org.uk/public/news/-national-report-dignity-and-nutrition-review-published. Accessed 5 July 2012.

30. Delmonthe, T., We need to talk about nursing. *BMJ*, 2011; 342, 3416.

31. Chandratilake, M., McAleer, S., Gibson J., *et al.*, Medical professionalism: what does the public think? *Clinical Medicine*, 2010; 10, 364–369.

32. Medical professionalism in the new millennium: a physicians' charter. *The Lancet*, 2002; 359, 520–522.

33. Verzulli, R., Jacobs, R. and Goddard, M., Do hospitals respond to greater autonomy? Evidence from the English NHS. University of York Centre for Health Economics Research Paper 64, July 2011. http://www.york.ac.uk/media/che/documents/papers/researchpapers/RP64_Foundation_Trusts.pdf. Accessed 5 July 2012.

34. Coiera, E., Why systems reforms makes health reforms so difficult. *BMJ*, 2011; 343, 27–29.

35. Jenkins, M., We need leaders, not leadership fads. *BMJ*, 2011; 342, d2552.

36. Academy of Medical Sciences, Clinical academic medicine in jeopardy: recommendations for change. June 2002. http://www.acmedsci.ac.uk/p99puid25.html. Accessed 5 July 2012.

37. Sheridan, D., Reversing the decline of academic medicine in Europe. *The Lancet*, 2006; 367, 1698–1701.

38. Wellcome Trust, Wellcome Trust calls for clearer vision for NHS reform. 20 May 2011. http://www.wellcome.ac.uk/news/media-office/press-releases/2011/WTVM051291.htm. Accessed 5 July 2012.

39. McCulloch, P., How to improve surgical research. *BMJ*, 2011; 343, 106.

40. Kmietowicz, Z., Health bill should include commitment to support medical research, say research leaders. *BMJ*, 2011; 342, d3196.

41. Keehan, S.P., Sisko, A.M., Truffer, C.J., *et al.*, National health spending projections through 2020: economic recovery and reform drive faster spending growth. *Health Affairs*, 2011; 30, 1594–1605.

42. Falcone, B.E. and Satiani, B., Physician as hospital chief executive officer. *Vascular and Endovascular Surgery*, 2008; 42, 88–94.
43. Darzi, A., A time for revolutions and the role of physicians in health care reform. *N. Engl. J. Med.*, 2009; 361, e8.
44. Gunderman, R. and Kanter, S.L., Educating physicians to lead hospitals. *Academic Medicine*, 2009; 84, 1348–1351.
45. Goodall, A.H., Physician-leaders and hospital performance: is there an association? *Social Science and Medicine*, 2011; doi:10.1016/j.socscimed.2011.06.025.
46. Horton, R., The doctor's role in advocacy. *The Lancet*, 2002; 359, 458.

7

The Global Demographic Challenge: The Role of Medical Science

All generations face challenges unique to their time in history. Perhaps our time will be remembered as a period of rapid advancement in science and technology on the one hand, and on the other, one which posed great global challenges. Of these challenges, the threat of global warming and the linked issue of human population growth are certainly unique in human history. Consumption of energy and the world's resources in general has never been greater and on a global scale never more unequal. Medical science too has advanced greatly during the past century and thereby contributed to the increased life expectancy we now enjoy. In doing so, it has also contributed to the global demographic challenges we now face. Advances in communication and transport have made the world a smaller place; for good or ill, the global village is here to stay, at least for the duration of our current civilisation. Globalisation is most frequently thought of in economic terms, however its impact on health in recent times has been a powerful reminder of its wider consequences. Two examples serve to illustrate this. The rapid spread of HIV/AIDs and the outbreak of SARS (severe acute respiratory syndrome) in 2003 demonstrated the ease with which viruses can adapt to our modern lifestyles. Travelling silently with their hosts, they have the potential to cross continents within hours and rapidly unleash global epidemics we would struggle to contain. Perhaps the present period will be remembered as the time in which globalisation occurred and when health too became a shared global concern. Significant advances have been made during the past two decades in understanding the threats to global health and the factors that underlie them, and progress has also been made in meeting them. Medical science has contributed to this and has much to offer in the future.

Population Growth and Global Health

The world's population today is close to 7 billion. It has increased from 2.5 billion in 1950 and is projected to reach 9.3 billion by 2100,[1] although UN projections vary considerably depending on fertility rates during the coming century. The projected global population estimate of 9.3 billion for 2100 is based on a medium fertility rate applied as a global average. Currently, 42% of the world's population lives in low fertility countries, that is, in countries where on average not enough female children are born to ensure that each woman is replaced by a daughter who survives to pro-creation age. Another 40% live in medium fertility countries in which each woman is replaced by between 1 and 1.5 daughters on average, and 18% live in high fertility countries in which each woman is replaced by more than 1.5 daughters. Population growth will therefore vary greatly between countries depending on local fertility rates. Countries with the highest fertility rates will experience continued population growth throughout the coming century, whereas growth in those countries with low and medium rates will peak around 2030 and 2060 respectively and decline thereafter (Figure 7.1).

Average longevity of the world's population has increased from around 45 years in 1950 to 68 years in 2009 and is expected to increase further to 75 years by 2050. Global fertility has declined from 4.9 births per woman in 1950 to 2.6 births in 2005–2010 and is expected to decline further to 2 births by 2050 (Figure 7.2). These average global figures conceal striking differences between regions. In more developed countries fertility is already well below replacement levels, whereas in the least developed countries it remains high at 4.5 children per woman. The combination of declining fertility and increasing longevity, known as the demographic transition, is also causing a dramatic aging of the world's population. For example, the percentage of people aged 60 and over increased from 8% in 1950 to 11% in 2009 and is expected to increase further to 22% by 2050

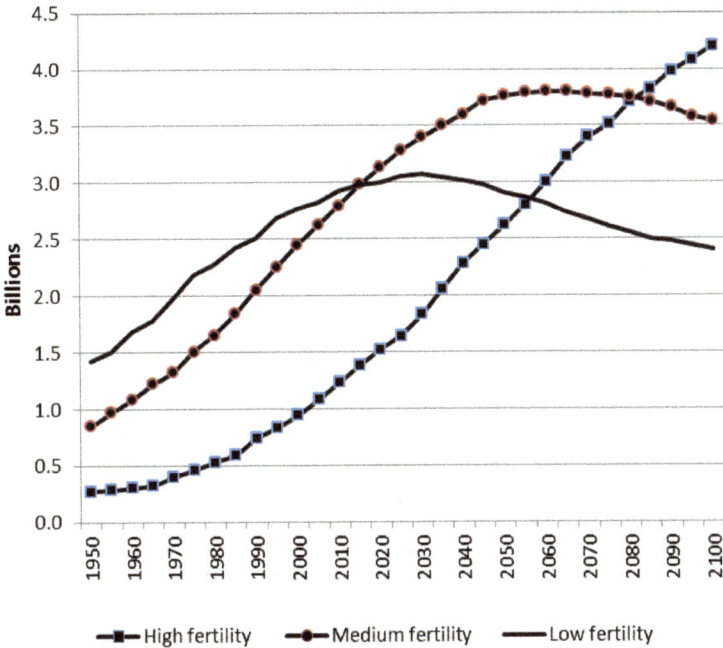

Figure 7.1. Changes in population from 1950 to 2010 and projected to 2100 for countries grouped by fertility rates. About 42% of the world's population live in low fertility countries, 40% in medium fertility countries and 18% in high fertility countries. Populations will peak around 2030 in those with low fertility rates and at 2060 in those with intermediate rates, but will continue to grow in those with high fertility rates. (Based on data from the United Nations World Population Prospects 2010 revision.[1])

(Figure 7.3). This aging process is most marked in high-income countries where fertility is lower and longevity greater. Thus, in 2009 the median ages of populations living in high-, middle- and low-income countries were 40, 26 and 20 years respectively, and these ages are expected to continue to rise to around 46, 37 and 30 years respectively by 2050 (Figure 7.4).

Demographic Transition

These changes in demography are both dramatic and unique; never before in human history, have people aged 65 and over outnumbered children under the age of five. Such changes will have profound effects on every aspect of our lives, including human health, family structures, patterns of

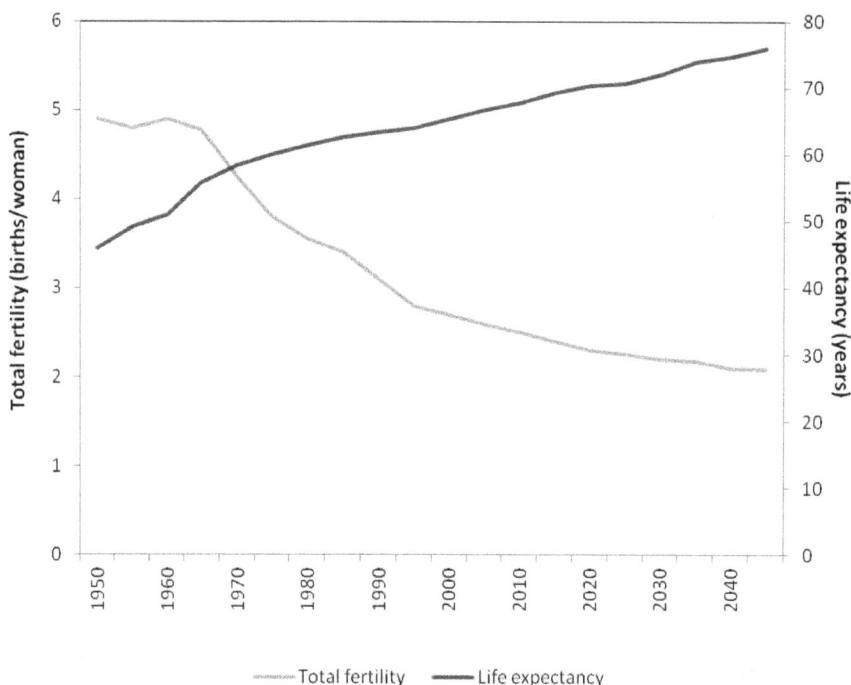

Figure 7.2. Global fertility rates and life expectancy between 1950 and 2009 and projected to 2050. The global demographic transition is illustrated by concomitant decline in fertility and increased life expectancy. (Based on data from the United Nations World Population Prospects 2010 revision.[1])

work and our economies. Provision of health care will also face many challenges as a result, and so too will the priorities and expectations of medical science. An immediate health consequence of the demographic transition is the reduction in the ratio of older to younger people, known as the support ratio. This is illustrated by the decline in the ratio of persons aged between 15 and 64 years to those aged 65 and over. The ratio shrank from 12:1 in 1950 to 9:1 in 2009, and is expected to fall further to just 4:1 by 2050 (Figure 7.5). Such changes indicate that in the future there will be fewer younger people available to support the elderly. The impact of the demographic transition is also compounded by the fact that life expectancy is longer in women than in men in all regions of the world. This results in a gender gap among older populations. Thus, in 2009, equal numbers of men and women comprised the world's population aged 40–49 years, but of

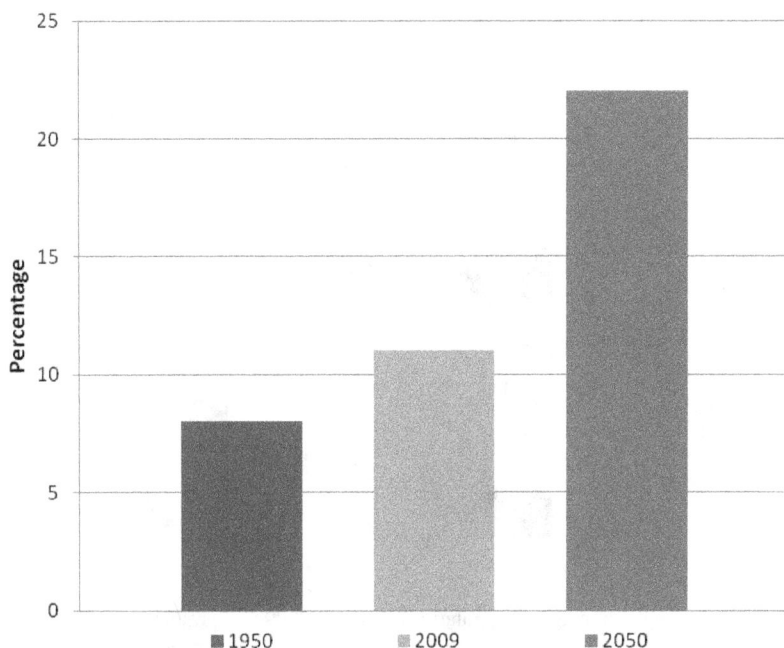

Figure 7.3. The percentage of the world population over 60 in 1950, 2009 and projected for 2050. The world population has aged dramatically and will continue to do so in the foreseeable future, due to a combination of declining fertility and increased life expectancy. (Based on data from the United Nations World Population Prospects 2010 revision.[1])

the population aged over 49 more were women, comprising 54% of people over 60 years, 63% over 80 years and 80% over 100 years (Figure 7.6). This gender difference is also most marked in high-income countries, where life expectancy also differs most between the sexes. Europe at present has the lowest sex ratio, with just 70 men per 100 women among people over 60, and 46 men per 100 women among people 80 and over. A further consequence of this gender age gap is a marked difference in the proportion of men and women with spouses. Thus globally, 80% of men aged 60 and over are married compared with just 48% of women.

Changes in the Burden of Disease

The Western world experienced marked improvement in life expectancy during the 20th century. Reductions in childhood mortality and infectious

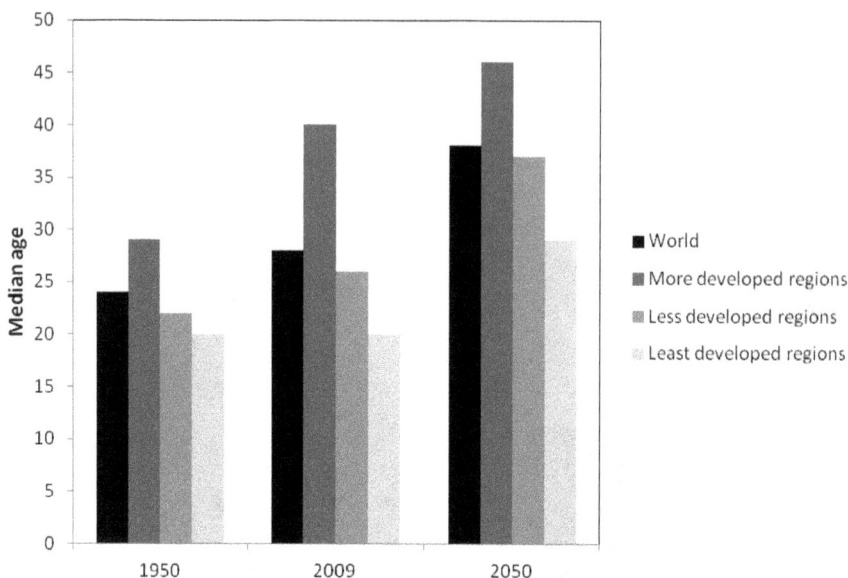

Figure 7.4.   The median age of populations in 1950, 2009 and projected for 2050 for the world and for regions based on economic status. Global aging is occurring in all regions, but is most marked in more developed countries. (Based on data from the United Nations World Population Prospects 2010 revision.[1])

diseases as well as the introduction of treatment and prevention of adult diseases, particularly cardiovascular disease, were major contributions to this improvement. Less-developed countries have continued to carry a heavy burden of disease. For example, in 2001, 19% of all deaths world-wide occurred in children and 99% of these children lived in low- and middle-income countries.[2] In 2001 in Sub-Saharan Africa and South Asia respectively, 80% and 60% of deaths in children under the age of five were due to infections and diarrhoeal disease. Globally, about a third of all deaths were attributable to communicable diseases, maternal and birth related conditions and nutritional deficiency. It is clear that these prevent-able conditions continue to exact a heavy toll in less-developed countries and this will require on-going effort in the years ahead. Nevertheless, the global pattern of disease burden has changed markedly in recent decades. Deaths in children under the age of five, although still severe, have fallen globally and in all regions of the world. With the exception of Sub-Saharan Africa, East Asia and the Pacific, where the reductions were between 9%

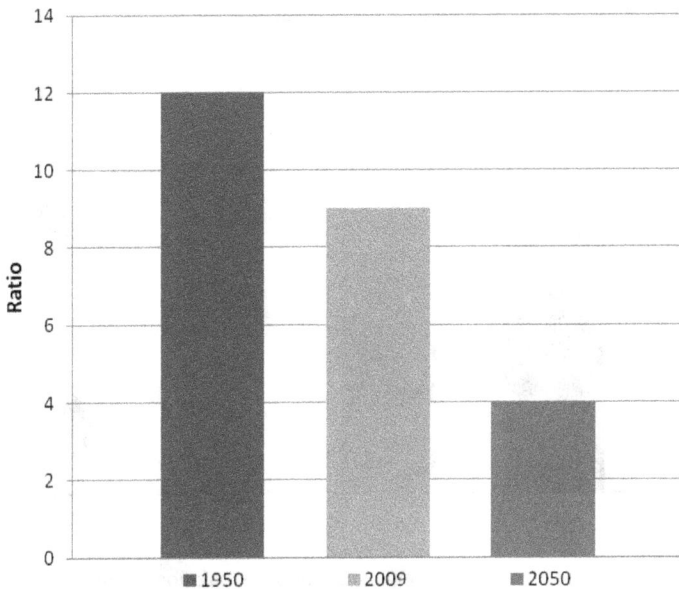

Figure 7.5.   The ratio of persons aged 15 to 64 to those aged 65 and over, known as the support ratio, in 1950, 2009 and projected for 2050. By 2050 the support ratio is projected to be just one third of what it was in 1950, indicating that in the future fewer younger people will be available to support those who are older. (Based on data from the United Nations World Population Prospects 2010 revision.[1])

and 27%, the global fall was more than 30%.[2] This has resulted from better nutrition, living conditions and health care. A second major change has been the decline in infectious diseases. Here, the picture is complicated by the sharp increase in deaths from HIV/AIDs, particularly in Sub-Saharan Africa, while other communicable diseases have declined. Thus, the age at which people die or become disabled in any population increases when health care improves and this also changes the conditions they are likely to suffer from, since many diseases are age related. For example, in 2001 in low- and middle-income countries 21% of deaths occurred among people aged 60 and over compared with 51% in high-income countries.[3] These changes, together with the increasing global life expectancy, have increased the importance of non-communicable diseases (NCDs), which in 2002 accounted for 44% and 54% of all deaths in low- to middle-income and high-income countries respectively, and which are projected to increase to 54% and 89% respectively by 2030.[3]

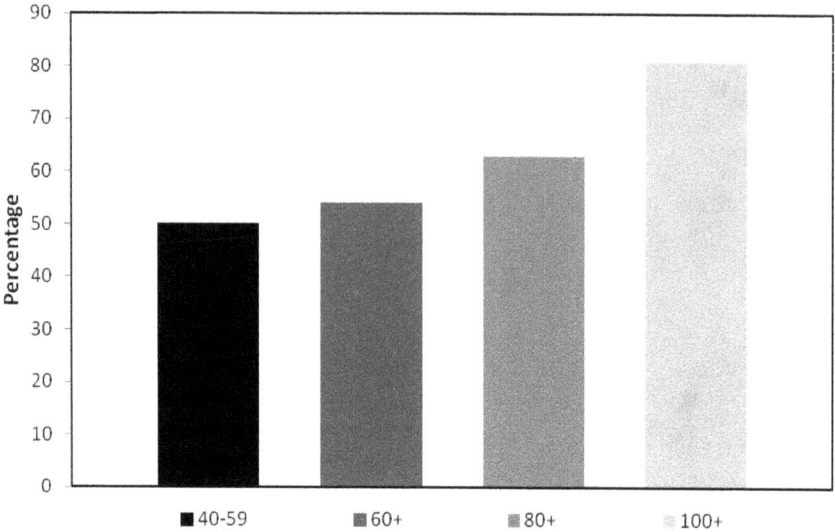

Figure 7.6. The percentage of women in the world's population grouped by age in 2009. Women make up a progressively greater part of the total with increasing age, so that among those over 80 years 63% are female. (Based on data from the United Nations World Population Prospects 2010 revision.[1])

Projected Trends in Disease Burden

As the demographic changes seen over the past several decades are set to continue, so too can we expect that the global patterns of diseases will continue to change. As people in all regions of the world are expected to live longer, an increasing number of deaths will occur later in life, and this has led to a projected increase in deaths due to NCDs from 59% in 2002 to 69% by 2030.[4] Communicable diseases are expected to decline, with the exception of HIV/AIDs which will continue to increase at a rate depending on the effectiveness of the current rollout of antiretroviral drugs and availability of a vaccine. Risk factors for chronic diseases will also play an important roll. For example, tobacco use is expected to cause 50% more deaths than HIV/AIDs in 2015 and 10% of all deaths globally.[3] Hypertension and diabetes are both major risk factors for cardiovascular disease. Hypertension is currently the most important risk factor globally[2] and will increase in all regions as populations age. In 2000, 171 million people globally were estimated to have diabetes and this figure is projected to increase to 366 million by 2030, based simply on projected trends in longevity. But the current epidemic of obesity will add substantially to this increase.

Responding to the Health Effects of Demographic Change

As discussed in Chapter 3, substantial progress has been made in meeting the challenge posed by HIV/AIDs and other infectious diseases. Infectious diseases are declining and significant progress has been made in fighting HIV/AIDs in most regions, Sub-Saharan Africa, East Asia and the Pacific being the exceptions. The achievements of the campaigns which galvanised public opinion and politicians in order to drive the political process that eventually released the substantial funding needed to mount this effort have been widely and rightly acknowledged. With the benefit of hindsight however two main criticisms of these efforts can be made. First, the effort was not sufficiently focused on the breadth of strategies needed to implement solutions most efficiently. It is now clear, for example, that although highly successful in driving down the cost of antiretroviral drugs to make them more widely available in less-developed countries, far too little attention was given to the logistics of delivering them to patients efficiently. Failure to address the problem of inadequate primary care staff, mainly nurses and support staff, continues to limit the effectiveness of investments in these countries.[6] More importantly, however, the shear success of the campaign is now seen to have heavily skewed funding of global health needs to the detriment of non-communicable diseases.[7,8]

The Era of Non-Communicable Diseases

The economic consequences of aging populations around the world have pressed all governments to focus on health care costs, which are expected to increase sharply. In EU countries, for example, health costs are estimated to rise by 15–40% in order to maintain current levels of provision.[9] In the developing world too, it is now being recognised that NCDs, having been neglected for years, will represent the greatest health burden in the decades ahead.[10] The UN held a High-level Meeting with heads of state

in September 2011 to develop strategies for tackling NCDs. In anticipa-
tion, advocacy groups put forward priority lists in the hope of influencing
the outcome of this discussion.[10–15] The lists focused on prevention by
introducing tobacco control, reducing poverty and illiteracy, and promoting healthy lifestyles through better diets and physical activity. However
disquiet has already been raised about a lack of attention to the means
of delivering better care, particularly in human resources.[15] Failure to
address the lack of adequate primary care risks repeating the subopti-
mal implementation and return on investment seen with the HIV/AIDs
campaign.[5]

It is beyond doubt that simple, inexpensive measures have been well
established in developed countries for preventing disability and death
from chronic diseases such as ischaemic heart disease, chronic bronchitis
and emphysema. Application of these measures at national and international levels in less-developed countries will be most effective in meeting
the global challenge of NCDs. Public health and social science have taken
the leading role in this, as they have for most of the advocacy of policy
recommendations for tackling this neglected and pressing issue.[7,10–15]
Added to this is the general tendency for advocates to see solutions to
problems in terms of their own expertise. Thus, fundraisers tend to see
mobilising resources as the key issue; politicians see creating the necessary political framework as the primary goal, and so on. The danger of this
is that the solutions arrived at may not integrate all of the available
resources needed to best meet the challenges. Failure to address the provision of the human resources needed to deliver the strategy for preventing
and treating HIV/AIDs illustrates this well. A further striking example of
how priorities can be skewed has been the neglect of chronic medical
conditions such as hypertension in the global health agenda. Despite the
fact that simple and inexpensive medicines to treat hypertension have
been widely available for many years, their use has frequently been
ignored, in contrast to the immense and highly successful campaign
to make antiretroviral medicines available for victims of HIV/AIDS.
For example, the WHO report World Health Statistics 2011[16] runs to
170 pages and includes a substantial section on risk factors for NCDs, but
does not even mention 'hypertension' or 'high blood pressure', one of the
major risk factors for premature death worldwide. This continuing neglect

of NCDs in such a recent report is extremely disappointing, but it gives a glimpse into the prevailing attitudes which perhaps explains why this area has been neglected for so long. It may in part reflect the traditional view that NCDs occur predominantly in Western countries and also that, given the size of the challenge and the proven effectiveness of lifestyle measures, medicines and research are low priorities. But the time when such views were justified is long gone. NCDs currently account for between 80% and 90% of deaths annually in low- and middle-income countries.[17] They kill more people in poorer than in richer countries (Figure 7.7), and in all age

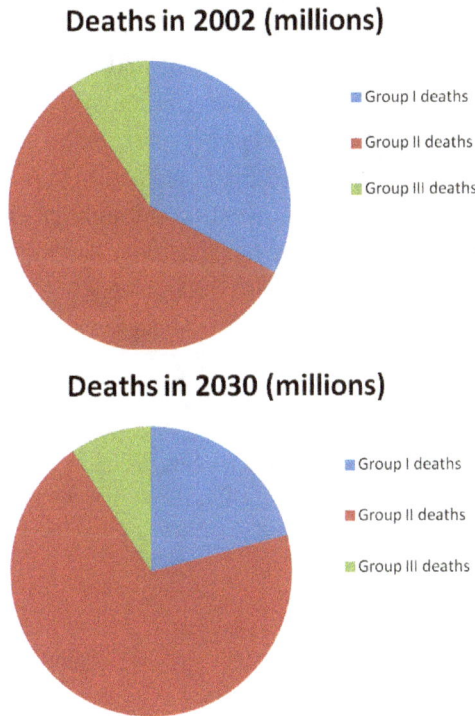

Deaths in 2002 (millions)

- Group I deaths
- Group II deaths
- Group III deaths

Deaths in 2030 (millions)

- Group I deaths
- Group II deaths
- Group III deaths

Figure 7.7. Deaths in 2002 and projected for 2030 based on group cause. Group I: HIV/AIDS, perinatal, respiratory infections and infections excluding HIV/AIDs. Group II: cardiovascular, cancer, respiratory and digestive conditions. Group III: violence and war, falls and road traffic accidents. Demographic changes and improvements in child health will result in major changes in the leading causes of death. Deaths due to communicable diseases, with the exception of HIV/AIDs will decline, but chronic diseases will kill many more people. (After Mathers *et al.*[4])

groups (Figure 7.8). In addition, the estimated increase in cancer deaths in 2030 compared with 2009 will be greater in low-income (82%) and middle-income (70%) countries than in high-income countries (40%).[4]

Meanwhile, given the growing awareness of the magnitude of this long neglected problem, the UN proposed a High-level Meeting of the General Assembly on the Prevention and Control of Non-communicable Diseases in September 2011.[18] The political declaration which resulted from this[19] made clear that NCDs are now recognised as a serious threat to global health, noting 'with profound concern' that an estimated 36 million of 57 million global deaths were due to NCDs in 2008. It was also declared that NCDs threaten economic development throughout the world and constitute one of the major challenges of the twenty first century. These results recognise the scale of the problem and the adverse impact that NCDs have on economic development, particularly in poorer countries. They also accept that NCDs are largely preventable through relatively simple and inexpensive measures.[19] Proposed action to radically reduce the burden of NCDs is built around prevention through the control of tobacco use, improving diets, promoting physical activity and reducing the harmful effects of alcohol. The hearing also recognised the importance of the eradication of illiteracy as well as fostering greater gender equality and

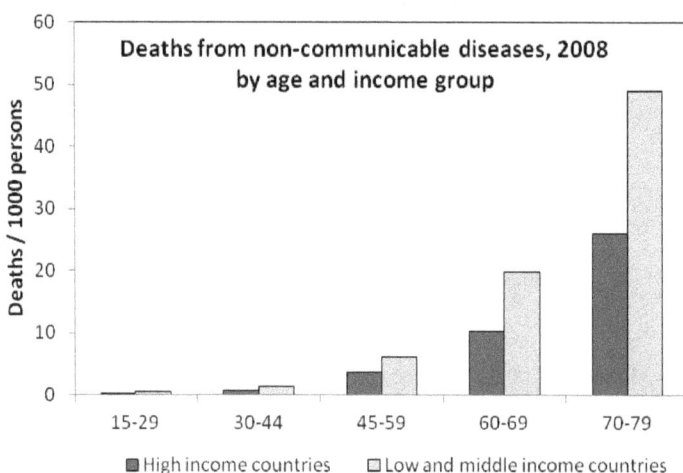

Figure 7.8. Deaths from non-communicable diseases by age and region income group. (Based on data from the United Nations World Population Prospects 2010 revision.[17])

empowering women in order to implement prevention strategies. The hearing also recommended that health care services should be developed to treat common high-risk conditions and that effective medicines be made available. Whether these deliberations will translate into effective action at a time of economic recession remains to be seen, but the challenge has been laid down and the action that follows will be watched by many.

Medical Science and Global Burden of Non-Communicable Disease

In contrast to the impressive energy that has been poured into the fight against HIV/AIDs, the scientific response to the global burden of chronic NCDs has been weak. Submissions to the UN have little to say about specific research or medical science in dealing with NCDs apart from the need for continued monitoring of their prevalence and the involvement of academia. An earlier report from the WHO was largely dismissive of what medical science could offer to combat many of the chronic diseases that are now known to carry the most severe burden globally.[20] At least, and to its credit, the recent UN preparatory work has now recognised the importance of integrated solutions, setting up adequate health care delivery systems and promoting research.[17] Does medical science have much to offer in meeting the global challenge of NCDs? The answer to this depends on whether we take a short- or long-term view of the challenge.

'Quick Wins' and Long-Term Solutions

Simple lifestyle measures, such as reducing tobacco and salt consumption, reducing weight, increasing physical activity and improving diets, can mitigate the impact of NCDs. Understandably this is the approach recommended by public health experts and has the added attraction of achieving rapid results.[21] Identifying and prioritising efforts that will bring about 'quick wins' is understandable. Doing what is possible now is a strategy that makes perfect sense, but advances in medicine have always been made by striving to do better. In considering what medical science can offer in meeting the global challenge of NCDs, I have chosen hypertension as an example, but many other such conditions would serve equally well.

Hypertension is now the world's largest risk factor for death, accounting for almost 8 million in 2008, and the second largest risk factor in terms of disability.[3] It has a global prevalence of around 40%, but is higher in lower-income countries. High cholesterol is the third largest risk factor for death and the fifth for disability.[3] It is undoubtedly the case that other factors, such as being overweight, having a poor diet and smoking, all contribute to the adverse effect of hypertension and high cholesterol, but even allowing for such factors hypertension and high cholesterol remain by far the most important contributors to ischaemic heart disease and stroke.

Bearing in mind the prevalence of hypertension and its consequences for global health, it is astonishing how little we know about its underlying causes. It can be diagnosed easily by simple measurement, but we know remarkably little about what initiates it, how it progresses during life or what events may precede its development. It has been known for decades that blood pressure tends to increase with age and this has been attributed to the loss of elasticity of blood vessels, commonly known as the 'hardening of arteries'. Recent evidence based on new scanning technology that allows the stiffness of arteries to be measured non-invasively has demonstrated that the hardening process begins in the thirties and is accompanied by increases in blood pressure.[22] This implies that the development of high blood pressure is related to changes in the circulation that begin much earlier than when it is usually detected by simple measurement. This takes us closer to an understanding of the problem in two important ways. Firstly, it provides us with methods and informs us where to look to try to understand the origins of the physical changes that lead to high blood pressure. Secondly, it provides a means to find ways to prevent these early changes and thereby prevent the eventual development of hypertension.

I have no doubt that the disturbances in circulation which cause hypertension will one day be unravelled. The great breakthrough in understanding how blood vessels regulate flow, for which Robert Furchgott received the Nobel Prize in 1998, may be the key to this. Yet this and other rich seams remain relatively unexplored and almost forgotten. Instead we are fascinated by molecular and genetic technology which struggles to deliver any tangible clinical benefits. Considering that hypertension has a global prevalence of 40% among adults, the immensity of the task of treating even a fraction of those suffering from its effects is surely daunting. Even allowing that effective and very low cost treatments are available, the benefit of research to better understand the causes of hypertension and how to prevent it seems abundantly clear. Yet this condition struggles for attention in the race for quick-fix solutions and immediate results.[20] A similar case can be made in relation to diabetes, the global prevalence of which is projected to increase from 2.4% to 4.4% by 2030, while the number of people with the condition will rise from 170 million in 2000 to 360 million by 2030,[5] based on projected aging and urbanisation patterns.[23] This study did not include the impact of the current global epidemic of obesity, and is therefore likely to be a significant underestimate. Once again, lifestyle measures such as weight reduction and healthier diets would be of great benefit. But there is also an urgent need to understand the links between glucose metabolism and the circulatory changes which lead to high blood pressure, stroke and ischaemic heart disease.

Medical research has contributed greatly to understanding the problems and challenges of global health. Indeed it was careful research which led to a better understanding of global demographic changes and their impact on global health and the distribution of disease. It was also high-quality research which revealed the current inequity of health care and the neglect of non-communicable diseases now being addressed. Furthermore, all of the prevention strategies and treatments we now take for granted arose from advances in medical science, and if we persist in searching for them future discoveries will undoubtedly lead to new and better ways to meet the challenges we now face. Our recent history tells us that we will face many new challenges to both regional and global health in the future and it is equally certain that our capacity for medical science will be crucial in confronting them. We can begin by recognising that medical science has much to offer in combating the global burden of NCDs. It has been effective in defining the extent of the challenge, but that is just a start. We also need a programme of science to find more effective diagnostic methods and treatments.

Medical Demographics

Demographic changes affecting health workers are a very small part of the global picture, but they too have an important impact on health. As early as 1978 the worldwide migration of physicians and nurses predominantly from poor to rich countries was recognised as a major contributor to global health inequity.[24] In 1972, 6% (140,000) of the world's physicians worked in countries other than the ones in which they were born, and of these three-quarters were in just three rich countries: the US, UK and Canada. The main donor countries were India, Pakistan and Sri Lanka. Loss of health workers is a serious issue for many less-developed countries, but particularly for those in Sub-Saharan Africa where the workforce has been seriously depleted due in part to the HIV/AIDs epidemic, but also migration. For example, the UK is a major recipient of health workers from poor countries with about 10–15% of nurses recruited from abroad between 1989 and 1996. This figure increased to 50% by 2002, with a corresponding reduction in those recruited from within the UK.[25] Furthermore, doctors recruited from outside the EU comprised 39% of medical trainees in the UK in 2006. One-fifth of African-born physicians (65,000 medics) migrate to developed countries within five years of qualifying[26] and more than a third of medical school faculty positions in Africa are vacant. As a result, the medical workforce in Africa is not sufficient to distribute and monitor treatment, limiting the impact of funds released by international donors to mitigate the HIV/AIDS epidemic. There are several reasons for worker migration but the overriding factors appear to be economic. Thus, the number of physicians available per 10,000 population correlates closely with a country's per capita GDP. Migration also responds to economic forces; countries with low GDP are losing doctors to those with high GDP.[24] It is accepted that donor countries gain certain advantages as a result of migration, such as repatriation of remittances and skills gained. This perception appears to have masked the much greater losses to donor countries that may contribute to forestalling the change of attitude needed to reverse the problem.

Lack of health workers is now recognised as a critical factor that is hindering health care in low-income countries, and consequently their economic development.[27] The key to reversing this is developing medical education and research capacity in those countries by funding research that is based and carried out locally, and building the infrastructure where it is lacking. There are signs that this approach is now being adopted through the Medical Education Partnership Initiative (MEPI) in the US[27] and in calls for equitable research collaborations.[28] It will be crucial that the UN also grasps this issue in its response to the burden of NCDs.

Gender Demographics in Medicine

Gender inequity is by far the most frequently discussed issue in medical demographics in recent years. Following calls for gender equity in the allocation of places in medical schools, changes were implemented in the UK which resulted in female entry rising from 24% in 1960 to 57% in 2007.[29] Similar changes leading to equality of entry have taken place in most Western countries. Even allowing that more time would be needed to translate this to equality at senior levels in the profession, female promotion has been slow. For example, in 1995 in the US, 83% of men had achieved associate or full professor rank after 11 years on medical faculties, compared with just 59% of women,[30] and similarly slow progress has been reported elsewhere.[29] This in part reflects a degree of social inertia or resistance to change in what has been described as a 'male dominated institution', which may lack the ability to examine the 'gender dimensions of its operations and values'.[31] However, wider underlying social and family conditions are also likely to play a role by encouraging more women than men to work part-time and to choose specialties that make this possible, but which may be less likely to lead to rapid promotion. Thus while achieving gender equality in access to medical school was remarkably swift and uncontroversial, progress has been slower at higher ranks in the profession. One concern was raised in 2004 that increasing numbers of women in medicine might weaken the profession's status and influence, citing the high proportion of women in teaching and in medicine in Russia as examples of professions with little influence.[32]

Maintaining the integrity of medical professionalism is certainly important at a time when the way medicine is being practised is undergoing change. As discussed in Chapter 6, the organisation of health care has undergone, and continues to undergo, rapid and repeated attempts at reform, often causing great upheaval. The profession has recognised the critical importance of maintaining and passing on to future generations its professional legacy through this period of change. It is undoubtedly the case that further reorganisation of health care provision will be needed to properly accommodate the aspirations of female doctors and their wish to continue to manage their family commitments. The issue, it seems to me, is not whether women can make doctors of equal standing with men; that is a given. What matters is ensuring that they have access to the necessary training and opportunities to allow them to rise to senior levels in medicine in a manner that recognises and respects their professionalism. Women must not be suborned into part-time lower-grade staff positions with less influence than men, but must be recognised as full equals to their male counterparts, working not in a kind of gender competition, but together, in support of patients and the profession as a whole.

A much greater and enduring inequity in medicine has been the inability to narrow the gap between socio-economic groups in medical school entry and in the profession as a whole.[33] Hopes that this could be addressed by widening the entry to medical schools in the UK to under-represented socio-economic groups have met with disappointment.[34] What is equally disappointing is the apparent lack of interest and willingness to address this issue more rigorously in order to reverse one of our most serious inequalities.

Highly talented campaigners have achieved remarkable progress in recent decades in tackling challenges such as HIV/AIDs, global health inequality and gender inequality in medicine. It is important that in focusing attention on the chosen cause, other equally important needs are not marginalised and disadvantaged.

Summary and Conclusions

Globalisation and changes in demographics have had a profound impact on health. Epidemics that would have been contained in former times can now have a global reach in mere days, and we are more aware than ever before of the health of the world's population as well as its inequalities. Increasing longevity and decreasing fertility have occurred in most regions of the world and have resulted in major demographic changes. For the first time in human history people aged 65 and over will soon outnumber children under five.

Demographic changes have also affected health care. Migration of health workers from low- to high-income countries has depleted the workforce in many countries and is now seen as a major obstacle, particularly in Sub-Saharan Africa, in efforts to treat patients with HIV/AIDs. Gender inequality among doctors has been reversed at the medical school level and among juniors in training, but is more resistant to change at senior levels. In contrast, little progress has been made in reversing social inequalities among doctors.

Substantial reductions in infant mortality and communicable diseases have been achieved in all regions. This is true also for HIV/AIDs, with the notable exception of countries in Sub-Saharan Africa, East Asia and the Pacific. As a result, the major causes of global ill-health are now chronic non-communicable diseases, which until recently have been neglected. Efforts are now being made to address this challenge with a new UN campaign. At present, most of the proposed interventions to reduce non-communicable diseases appear to be focused on social measures, with reduction in tobacco consumption and salt intake, anti-obesity measures and increased physical exercise as key elements.

Medical science led the way in defining the extent of this health burden and it has a great deal to offer in confronting it. Better understanding of high-risk conditions such as hypertension, the links between diabetes and being overweight, and finding much better treatments and preventive measures are needed and are well within the reach of medical science, if properly supported.

References

1. UN Department of Economic and Social Affairs, World population prospects 2010 revision. http://esa.un.org/wpp/unpp/panel_population.htm. Accessed 5 July 2012.
2. Lopez, A.D., Mathers, C.D., Ezzati M., *et al.*, Global and regional burden of disease and risk factors, 2001: systematic analysis of population health data. *The Lancet,* 2006; 367, 1747–1757.
3. Lopez, A.D., Mathers, C.D., Ezzati, M., *et al.* (Eds), *Global Burden of Disease and Risk Factors.* 2006. http://www.ncbi.nlm.nih.gov/books/NBK11812/. Accessed 5 July 2012.

4. Mathers, C.D. and Loncar, D., Projections of global mortality and burden of disease from 2002 to 2030. *PLoS Med,* 2006; 3(11), e442.

5. Wild, S., Roglic, G., Green, A., *et al.,* Global prevalence of diabetes: estimates for the year 2000 and projections for 2030. *Diabetes Care,* 2004; 27(5), 1047–1053.

6. Narasimhan, V., Brown, H., Pablos-Mendez, A., *et al.,* Responding to the global human resources crisis. *The Lancet,* 2004; 363, 1469–1472.

7. Stuckler, D., King, L., Robinson, H., *et al.,* WHO's budgetary allocations and burden of disease: a comparative analysis. *The Lancet,* 2008; 372, 9649.

8. Sheridan, D.J. and Heusch, G., Threats to the future of cardiovascular research. *The Lancet,* 2009; 373, 875–876.

9. European Commission, 2009 ageing report: economic and budgetary projections for the EU-27 member states (2008–2060). February 2009. http://ec.europa.eu/economy_finance/publications/publication14992_en.pdf. Accessed 5 July 2012.

10. Geneau, R., Stuckler, D., Stachenko, S., *et al.,* Raising the priority of preventing chronic diseases: a political process. *The Lancet,* 2010; 376, 1689–1698.

11. Beaglehole, R., Bonita, R., Horton, R., *et al.,* Priority actions for the non-communicable disease crisis. *The Lancet,* 2011; 377, 1438–1447.

12. Sridhar, D., Morrison, J.S. and Piot, P., Expectations for the United Nations High-level Meeting on non-communicable diseases. *Bull. World Health Organ.,* 2011; 89, 471.

13. Beaglehole, R., Bonita, R., Alleyne, G., *et al.,* UN High-level Meeting on non-communicable diseases: addressing four questions. *The Lancet,* 2011; 378, 449–455.

14. Alwan, A.D., Galea, G. and Stuckler, D., Development at risk: addressing non-communicable diseases at the United Nations High-level Meeting. *Bull. World Health Organ.,* 2011; 89, 546–546A.

15. Maher, D. and Ford, N., Action on non-communicable diseases: balancing priorities for prevention and care. *Bull. World Health Organ.,* 2011; 89, 547–547A.

16. WHO, World health statistics 2011. WHO, Geneva, 2011. http://www.who.int/gho/publications/world_health_statistics/en/index.html. Accessed 5 July 2012.

17. WHO, Global status report on non-communicable diseases 2010. April 2011. http://www.who.int/nmh/publications/ncd_report2010/en/. Accessed 5 July 2012.

18. UN General Assembly, United Nations preparatory papers ahead of High-level Meeting on non-communicable diseases held in September 2011. http://www.un.org/en/ga/president/65/issues/ncdiseases.shtml. Accessed 5 July 2012.

19. UN General Assembly, Prevention and control of non-communicable diseases: report of the Secretary-General. May 2011. http://www.un.org/ga/search/view_doc.asp?symbol=A/66/83&Lang=E. Accessed 5 July 2012.

20. Kaplan, W. and Laing, R., Priority medicines for Europe and the world. WHO report, November 2004. http://whqlibdoc.who.int/hq/2004/WHO_EDM_PAR_2004.7.pdf. Accessed 5 July 2012.

21. Capewell, S. and O'Flaherty, M., Rapid mortality falls after risk factor changes in populations. *The Lancet,* 2011; 378, 752–753.

22. Redheuil, A., Yu, W.C., Wu C.O., *et al.*, Reduced ascending aortic strain and distensibility: earliest manifestations of vascular aging in humans. *Hypertension*, 2010; 55, 319–326.

23. Hightower, J.D., Hightower, C.M., Vázquez, B.Y., *et al.*, Incident prediabetes/diabetes and blood pressure in urban and rural communities in the Democratic Republic of Congo. *Vasc. Health Risk Manag.*, 2011; 7, 483–489.

24. Mejia, A., Migration of physicians and nurses: a world wide picture. *Int. J. Epidemiology*, 1978; 7, 207–215.

25. Nursing and Midwifery Council, *NMC Annual Reports 2000–2003*. Nursing and Midwifery Council, London, 2003.

26. International Organization for Migration, *World Migration 2005*. International Organization for Migration, Geneva, 2005.

27. Collins, F.S., Glass, R.I., Whitescarver, J., *et al.*, Developing health workforce capacity in Africa. *Science,* 2010; 330, 1324–1325.

28. Crane, J., Scrambling for Africa? Universities and global health. *The Lancet,* 2011; 377, 1388–1389.

29. Royal College of Physicians, Women and medicine: the future. June 2009. http://bookshop.rcplondon.ac.uk/details.aspx?e=277. Accessed 5 July 2012.

30. Tesch, B.J., Wood, H.M., Helwig, A.L., *et al.*, Promotion of women physicians in academic medicine: glass ceiling or sticky floor? *JAMA*, 1995; 273, 1022–1025.

31. Reichenbach, L. and Brown, H., Gender and academic medicine: impacts on the health workforce. *BMJ*, 2004; 329, 792–795.

32. Hath, I., Women in medicine. *The Lancet*, 2004; 329, 412–413.

33. BMA Equal Opportunities Committee, Equality and diversity in UK medical schools. October 2009. http://www.bma.org.uk/-/media/Files/PDFs/Developing%20your%20career/Becoming%20a%20doctor/Equality%20diversity%20diversity%20in%20medical%20schools%202011.pdf. Accessed 5 July 2012.

34. Mathers, J., Sitch, A., Marsh, J.L., *et al.*, Widening access to medical education for under-represented socioeconomic groups: population based cross sectional analysis of UK data, 2002–6. *BMJ*, 2011; 342, d918. doi: 10.1136/bmj.d918.

8

Biomedical Science in Modern Economies: Innovation and Health

Since the industrial revolution science has been the engine of Western economies, providing the means for modern transport, rapid communication, better health and longer lives. We have come to rely on an almost automatic and steady flow of knowledge, inventions and innovations to develop 'the next big thing' to drive each new cycle of economic growth and employment. When economies are in recession we anxiously look for signs of recovery; we try to identify the key bottlenecks that are stalling progress and argue about policies and strategies to relieve them. Innovation, meaning changes to existing products or new ones that capture market share and boost sales and profits, has become the key to success. Replication of innovation fuels economic growth and creates employment. Much of our public discourse relates to social and political conditions that may hinder or promote it. Although the scientific discoveries which lead to innovations are usually acknowledged, they tend to be overshadowed by the entrepreneurial achievement in their development.[1] Economists, academics and cities compete in setting up 'centres of innovation' that will bring together the institutions needed to make this happen. The idea is that once a critical mass is reached, the innovation process will ignite spontaneously. A picture emerges in which ideas, concepts and knowledge arise by some reliable automatic process; we only need to grasp them and create the right conditions to turn them into products that will compete successfully in the market place.

Innovation

Seeking new and better ways to make things is clearly laudable, particularly if they are more efficient and use fewer material resources and less energy. Creating jobs is also desirable, especially in times of recession. At present, 'innovation' is widely considered the key to achieving both goals. But what do we mean by innovation? The word has a long been used to mean novelty, as seen when King Henry accuses Worcester of using novelty to decorate 'the garment of rebellion with some fine colour that may please the eye of fickle changelings and discontents, which gape and rub the elbow at the news of hurly burly innovation'.[2] It was not until the 20th century that the word took on the economic intent we are now so familiar with. In his classic work, *Business Cycles*,[3] Joseph Schumpeter used the word to define the taking of new ideas, knowledge or inventions into the economic process through the investment of capital to produce novel products and services. He pointed out that innovations sometimes occur as the result of an economic need, but at other times they actually generate a need. The motorcar is an example of this; there was no expressed need for such a vehicle prior to its introduction, but once it became available, demand followed. Similar examples have been powerful drivers of economies and explain why innovation is considered such a potent economic force. Like King Henry, some may have reservations that the 'next big thing' will turn out to be a trivial diversion, and wasteful if it is quickly overtaken by a following wave of innovation as product cycles get shorter and shorter, but today innovation is mostly viewed as a kind of economic genie that drives growth and prosperity.

Science, Invention and Innovation

Schumpeter saw a clear distinction between inventions and the process of innovation carried out by entrepreneurs, pointing out that innovation does not require any invention and inventions do not necessarily lead to any innovation. He placed a higher value on innovation, citing examples of inventions that may be known about for generations with little or no impact on society or the economy, but that when incorporated into an innovation may finally have a wide-ranging effect on both. He describes innovations as the result of planned ventures (what he called the 'volitional actions of businessmen'), in contrast to inventions which are more likely to arise by chance ('autonomously' or by 'happy accident', a result of what he described as 'personal aptitudes, primarily intellectual in the case of the inventor'). He stressed that there is no consistent interdependence between innovations and inventions and went on to describe the methods that lead to them as 'belonging to different spheres' and the social processes that produce them as being quite different. This view, that innovation is independent of invention and scientific knowledge, led Schumpeter to give much less credit to the role of science in the process of innovation. Later economists would take a different view, accepting that innovation is part of a much larger and complex process in which invention is often the first of several stages. James Allen, for example, distinguished six components in the innovation process,[4] including the creation of an idea and its development as well as organising investment to implement it, its construction and distribution. Nevertheless, the idea often persists that the business end of development is the key to success and is the limiting step that needs our attention. Headlines such as 'The next big thing won't happen on its own' and 'Entrepreneurs need more than just ideas'[5] appear to be straight out of Schumpeter's early and rather narrow views. It seems to me however, that innovation, invention and scientific knowledge are not only closely linked, but also interdependent, and that failure to recognise this and how the three concepts need to work together is at the root of problems faced by many industries, including biomedical science today, and I will return to this later.

Innovation and Economic Growth

It is almost impossible in the modern world to find an area of our lives which has not been influenced by innovation. Transport by air, railway and road have increased our mobility to an astonishing degree during the past century. As discussed in previous chapters, new medicines and surgical techniques have brought cures for many diseases and prolonged the lives of many of us. Communication has undergone a revolution with immense social and political consequences. Innovations in the domestic sphere have greatly improved the quality of home life. We have all seen and been touched by the positive effects of innovation. In economic terms, innovation has produced extraordinary levels of growth during the past century. We have seen completely new industries emerge based on the production of motorcars and aircraft and more recently staggering growth based around computers and communications equipment. Countries that have been able to participate in these developments have also experienced unprecedented economic growth and prosperity, which in turn has led to improved quality of life and health for their citizens. Innovation has indeed been at the heart of much of this success; it is hardly surprising therefore that we should regard sustaining it as a key factor for our continued wellbeing.

Adverse Effects of Innovation

In recent years, by associating innovation with industrial production and prosperity, it often appears that these concepts are linked automatically with economic benefit and our ability to compete in the global market place, to a degree that tends to overshadow other aspects of human endeavour. The principal reason for this, it seems to me, is a widely held view of innovation as part of a highly simplified economic model. The idea here is that the principle measures of success are market capture, sales and profit. It matters little how useful, or indeed harmful, an innovation is in this sense. As Everett Rogers pointed out, it is unimportant whether an innovation has any particular advantage over what it replaces, what matters is whether the individual perceives it to have an advantage.[6]

But there are two important reasons for taking a wider view of innovation. Firstly, innovations may be harmful as well as beneficial, and secondly, a broader view of how innovation works is needed to sustain its role. It is not difficult to find examples of harmful innovations. Antibiotics and tobacco have both been highly successful innovations in the economic sense, yet tobacco will kill 50% more people in the world than HIV/AIDs in 2015.[7] More generally, we now realise that untrammelled consumption of many innovations can have negative effects on society, such as air pollution, global warming and so on. Our perception of what appears advantageous may be misconceived, or we may be misled by marketing techniques. In other words, from a societal point of view it is far too simplistic to regard the short-term success of the sales department or share value as the ultimate measure of the success of an innovation. It may be that in some cases the costs resulting from the consumption of an innovation are so high or the risks involved so great that the enterprise may not be justified. Given our present understanding of the harmful effects of tobacco consumption, would it be considered an acceptable innovation today? Thus, it is clearly important to consider the overall value of innovations and how they are used in a broad context of human need.

Regulation of Innovation

Of course, if left untouched, one can see that adverse conditions induced by excessive consumption of any particular innovation would eventually self-correct since it would in time hinder further consumption; in other words, a point would arise when the effects of overuse might have a negative impact on the course of economic evolution itself, and this would force a change. For example, a continued rise in global temperature from excessive use of fossil fuels might have such deleterious effects that alternative sources of energy and more efficient converters would be sought. We can see this in action today as industries and governments endeavour to protect their future businesses and economics through political actions such as the Kyoto protocol. In this sense, it might be argued that economic evolution can be trusted to self-correct; this is a view that many economists seem to hold. Some might disagree on the basis that it is largely non-industrialists, such as independent scientists and governments, who are pressing for a reduction in greenhouse gas emissions. But this argument ignores the fact that much of our knowledge and understanding of global warming and carbon dioxide levels are dependent on our scientific institutions, which in turn are ultimately dependent on taxes raised from productive economies for support and funding. Some parts of our industries may not support actions proposed to reduce emissions of greenhouse gases, but the tax income they generate nevertheless contributes indirectly to actions proposed to do so.

Innovation and Health

The adverse impact some innovations have on health clearly shows that economically driven self-correction does not work. The cost in human lives of tobacco consumption is beyond doubt. In most Western countries this has forced governments to suppress tobacco consumption through taxation, thereby controlling its use. In one sense it could again be argued that this is an action generated by the economy itself since taxes raised from economic activity have supported the gathering of evidence on which the action is based; the economy might be said to have reacted because of the high economic costs involved. However, even if we accept the economic argument, the response it has generated has been far too inadequate and slow to prevent the global health catastrophe that continues to unfold. Furthermore, the response has been indifferent to health losses incurred beyond the borders of national economies, as exemplified by the fact that legislation in Western countries does not restrict tobacco companies resident there or their subsidiaries from actively creating markets in developing countries to replace those lost at home. Of course, as discussed in Chapter 7, we now have a new UN global response to non-communicable diseases, which proposes a worldwide strategy on tobacco. In so far as all of this activity is supported by and is dependent on economic activity, this approach might also be argued to be another example of economic self-correction. However, even if we accept this argument self-correction is evidently incapable of protecting human health.

Alcohol consumption also illustrates how tolerant many countries appear to be of the harmful effects of innovations for the sake of preserving the apparent economic benefits. Innovations in the promotion and sale of alcohol have achieved marked increases in consumption in recent years, and as a result illness attributable to the use of alcohol is now second only to tobacco in countries with established market economies.[8] Regulation has been shown to have been capable of curtailing excessive consumption in the past, and when implemented it appears to have been motivated largely by economic concerns, for example, the perceived threat of alcohol use to industrial productivity at the outbreak of the First World War in the UK. In recent times, deregulation in the UK has been associated with increased consumption and a marked rise in alcohol related illness; deaths from liver disease have more than doubled since 1986.[9] The cost to the NHS in the UK has also increased substantially, standing at around £3 billion in 2002,[10] but this is only around 5% of the costs to the wider society, estimated to be £55 billion.[11] Most professionals working with the consequences of this have little confidence in present moves to curtail alcohol consumption.[9] It may seem extraordinary that we are willing to accept such a high price in terms of loss of human health and the associated costs. The fact is however that as yet there is no evidence that the labour market or industrial production are being jeopardised by this rise in consumption. For as long as there is no evidence that alcohol harms productivity we appear to be willing to tolerate the costs involved in the name of preserving free choice and free trade. But anyone who deals with the health aspects of addictive substances such as tobacco, alcohol or illicit drugs knows that free choice is a poor defence against the harm they cause for most people who misuse them.

Mistrust of Innovations

One of the most striking paradoxes of the 21st century is a growing mistrust of innovations related to our health, despite the obvious fact that we have benefitted immensely from so many successful new treatments and diagnostic methods over the past century. Many people are concerned about possible harmful effects of vaccines and electromagnetic radiation from mobile phones and power lines, often despite available evidence to the contrary. As I write, the level of suspicion about genetically modified food among many members of the public seems so great that it is hard to imagine that any amount of evidence will be sufficient to allay their fears. Among health care professionals also, many appear concerned that innovations may be harmful by causing uncontrolled growth in expenditure, and that this needs to be controlled.[12] Similarly, mistrust due to fears of unforeseen harmful side-effects is also contributing to increased regulation and in turn increased drug development costs. In many of the above examples the issue is often more about mistrust than evidence of harm.

Many scientists believe that genetically modified food will prove no more harmful to human health than the selective breeding of grains for beneficial characteristics over past generations, and yet many members of the public remain mistrustful of it; the reason for this can be traced back to the perception that innovations are introduced primarily for the benefit of producers and shareholders and that public benefit is at best secondary. The irony here is that just as the success of an innovation depends on a public perception that it offers some advantage (even where there is none), so too the process of innovation can be hindered by a public perception that it carries undue risks (even where there is none or very little). Both positions seem to originate in a 'buyer beware' mentality and some instances in which the buyer has felt short-changed. The danger here is that public perception of risks associated with innovation in some industries, such as drug development, can lead to mistrust and demands for regulations that are not cost effective[13] and which ultimately can begin to inhibit innovation itself. As discussed in Chapter 5, this is an important issue facing the pharmaceutical industry and biomedical science today. Thus, a sense that innovations are driven by market imperatives while social or health priorities are secondary, or in some cases disadvantaged, is clearly detrimental. It leads to mistrust in the process of innovation specifically and in science in general that relates to the purpose of innovation rather than its products. As discussed in Chapter 3, surveys show that people are much more trustful of independent scientists than those who work for government agencies or certain industries, such as those concerned with nuclear power, genetically modified food and pharmaceuticals.[14] The tragedy here is that these concerns may not discriminate between innovations that would be of great benefit for society and those that may be harmful. This lack of discrimination also explains why this mistrust has proven so resistant to scientific evidence of safety since the problem is less about science and more about where it comes from and perceptions about its purpose. In the same way concerns about drug development may be less about a lack of evidence of safety and more about poor ethical standards in the pharmaceutical industry and some aggressive or illegal corporate policies. All of this mistrust ultimately arises from the perception that innovations are driven too much by short-term economic imperatives that are not always consistent with wider societal values and needs. There are some indicators that the economic damage inflicted by this short-term thinking is being recognised,[15] so perhaps we may be seeing the beginning of a redirection; if so, it looks like being a long, slow and painful process.

There is no doubt that Western economies have proved hugely successful in creating the wealth needed to develop and maintain stable societies and that they are immensely important for our future wellbeing. However, societies are more than just economies and people are more than just contributors to GDP. We need to protect and maintain our innovative capacity, but it cannot be sensible that we should regard the performance of our economy as the ultimate measure of our success as a society. Neither can it be right that we should consider the protection of all sectors of our economies, including those that have a negative impact on health, as our highest priority. By the same token, and as the tobacco and alcohol examples shows, it is evident that we cannot rely on the self-correcting mechanisms proposed by economic theory to protect other aspects of societal wellbeing, such as health. Ultimately damage to economies may lead to a change of direction and a return to growth. However economic cycles are not responsive to health needs which, as a result, can suffer catastrophic consequences if economies are allowed to 'self steer'.

Innovation in Biomedical Science

A further reason to take the wider view of innovation, as suggested by James Allen,[4] is the need to consider the factors required to sustain it. This matters particularly for medicine because of declining research productivity in the pharmaceutical industry. As discussed in Chapter 5, the industry has faced a sixfold increase in drug development costs since 1979.[16] The great wealth accumulated due to its successes in the 20th century has allowed the industry to meet these higher costs, but this will not be sustainable in the longer term. Some economists have argued to the contrary, that the problem can be overcome simply by demanding higher prices for new drugs coming onto the market, as occurred between the mid-1990s and 2003.[17] This is essentially the blockbuster model of drug development and although there have been some notable commercial successes, this model also contains serious weaknesses. It tends to narrow the focus of research to achieve 'the big hit' based on market opportunities and restricts the portfolio of treatments being developed, particularly for rare diseases and those which occur predominantly in low-income countries. It also increases the risk of failure for companies in search of a blockbuster drug if their drug fails to get approval. Furthermore, consumers and purchasers have already responded to rising drug costs by introducing value-based pricing,[18] whereby the value of drug sales relates more to health benefits rather than just development costs.

A Crisis in Pharmaceuticals

There is general agreement that the present model of drug development is not working and that the pharmaceutical industry is in crisis.[19–21] It is important therefore to consider what has gone so wrong and how to restore and sustain innovation in this vital industry. The crisis facing the industry is real and is largely one of research productivity.[21] One response has been an increase in mergers and acquisitions as large pharmaceutical companies simply buy up the pipelines of smaller rivals. But such opportunities are diminishing as the number of pipelines reduces. During the past two decades, several large pharmaceutical companies have moved their R&D investment to the US. This reflects a desire to be closer to the largest markets and also to the Food and Drug Administration, which regulates approval in the US. The possibility that research productivity is higher in the US has also been considered as a reason for these moves; however recent work suggests that declining research productivity is a global problem and is not confined to any particular region.[21] It therefore seems unlikely that regional differences in knowledge, skills or investment are significant contributing factors to research productivity, which is perhaps not surprising given the ease of cross-border flows of capital and labour.

Recent rapid developments in biomedical science have also been suggested to explain the decline in research productivity in drug development since it inevitably takes some time for new developments in science to be incorporated into new treatments. It has therefore been suggested that the present crisis in pharmaceuticals may only be temporary due to a lag phase in exploiting recent developments of molecular technology and genetics.[22] This may prove to be the case, but there are increasing concerns that recovery on this basis is still a distant prospect. Even if true, this premise rests on an assumption that the benefits of discoveries in biomedical science will flow primarily into medical advances. We might wish to think that this will happen since much of this work is funded from medical research budgets, however history has repeatedly shown the unpredictability of the route by which discoveries translate into useful innovations. At present we are already seeing dramatic advances, based on new technologies, in understanding human evolution and our genetic links to some of our predecessors, as well as in plant biology. It may therefore be that the lag phase is over and uses for recent biomedical discoveries are already emerging, but less in the form of new medicines than had been hoped.

Low Hanging Fruit and the Rush for Gold

Some have suggested that research efforts in the 20th century have simply exhausted the more easily-targeted therapeutic opportunities and that those remaining are more complex and require new technologies.[23,24] The idea here is that drug targets revealed by methods used in the 19th and 20th centuries, such as pharmacology and pathophysiology, have all been mined and that new and more complex methods are needed to replace them. The argument goes that there is a natural lag phase before the benefits of technical advances in biological sciences can be realised in terms of clinical applications. This is a popular view, but one that is difficult to confirm since it is always difficult to prove the absence of something. It certainly is true that a large proportion of biomedical science budgets in academia and in industry was transferred into molecular biology and genetics at the end of the 20th century. However there is no evidence that this occurred because previously-used methods had failed to deliver, rather it appears to have been motivated by the hope that these new and exciting areas would quickly uncover new opportunities. Hedge-fund managers, big pharma and grant funders all piled into the new technologies in a manner reminiscent of a 19th century gold rush. And there is no doubt that many new fundamental scientific discoveries have been made, but the results to date have been far less rewarding in terms of new treatments.

Science Reveals the Unexpected

What these new sciences have revealed is a new and immensely more complex picture of biology. For example, the human genome consists of approximately 24,000 genes, the functions of almost all of which are unknown. These functions will need to be clarified in order to understand their role in health and disease. This is an immense task which led to the creation of a new body of science known as functional genomics. Furthermore, the functions which genes control are often mediated by proteins, which are synthesised in the body based on the specific code of the genes concerned. The need to understand the roles played by these proteins has led to yet another new area of biology, proteomics. And the scale of numbers and the interactions involved has required the development of a new specialty of mathematics, informatics. Furthermore, interactions between individual genes and between the large numbers of proteins that mediate their functions are also far more complex than originally envisaged. Scientists now recognise that this complexity is, in itself, a major issue and are endeavouring to find new techniques to deal with it. The challenge facing scientists seeking new and better treatments for heart failure illustrates this well; here, the network of potentially interacting genes and molecules is now so great that new systems have had to be devised simply to manage them.[25]

It will be for historians in the future to unravel whether the large-scale flight from traditional fields of biomedical science, such as clinical science, pathophysiology, etc., was wise or whether it contributed to the decline in drug research productivity. Meanwhile, it is increasingly clear that the myriad of interacting processes that the new technologies are revealing will have to be understood in terms of their impact on living beings, and this will not be possible without some recourse to these classical approaches, even if their return appears under the guise of new names such as 'systems biology'.

Declining R&D Productivity and 'The Burden of Knowledge'

Declining R&D productivity is not confined to the biomedical science industry, but appears to be a general feature of advanced economies.

In fact, research productivity has been declining for several decades in many Western countries despite increasing investment in R&D. So perhaps the problems facing the pharmaceutical industry are simply another manifestation of this. For example, the ratio of patents to scientists and engineers in 1990 had fallen to around half the levels reported in 1970 in the US, UK, Germany and France.[23] The number of scientists and engineers in the US increased from 500,000 in 1965 to around 1 million in 1989, but the number of patents granted remained fairly constant; furthermore, per capita economic growth rates either remained constant or declined over the same period.[24] Economic models which included an assumed decline in R&D productivity over time best explain the observed economic behaviour.[24] In an attempt to explain this phenomenon, some have drawn attention to the possible negative impact of increasing knowledge on innovation. For example, industrial networks become more complex as technology advances[26] and this increasing complexity has been put forward to explain declining R&D productivity in developed countries. Others have pointed out that as knowledge accumulates, so do the educational demands faced by innovators. Increasing information also leads to specialisation and in turn to a greater reliance on teams to maintain a sufficient range of expertise. It has therefore been argued that innovation becomes more difficult and more costly[27] as knowledge grows.

There are several reasons why this hypothesis is unlikely to correct, particularly in science-based industries; indeed, new knowledge might be thought of as a critical factor that promotes innovation. Furthermore, humanity has been accumulating new knowledge throughout history and there is no evidence that this has been a gradually increasing barrier to innovation. Neither is there any evidence that the human capacity to hold knowledge has increased over time commensurate with the growth of knowledge, and periods spent in education has only increased in recent times. Humans appear to adapt to the emergence of new knowledge remarkably well, by packaging information into more easily managed arrangements. Indeed the process of doing so itself involves innovation. For example, the introduction of the microprocessor resulted from several advances in the development of silicon chips and integrated circuits. Anyone wishing to use one initially would have been required to understand the design of the circuit, the architecture of its central processor and memory, the instruction set it responded to and how it communicated with external devices. The level of education needed to achieve this would have restricted their use to small sections of science and industry. By building the information into mass-produced personal computers it has became widely available and accessible, a process that itself involved many successful innovations that have generated great wealth for some companies. In other words, humans manage the 'burden' of new knowledge as they have always done, by packaging collections of it into useful resources, such as tools and machines.

Knowledge to Promote Innovation

How then, and in what sense, could new knowledge be a hindrance to innovation? It is beyond question that the inventions and discoveries that led to the microprocessor produced a rapid succession of successful innovations resulting in the emergence of many successful companies. And yet, it is also clear that as knowledge continued to grow and microprocessor design became more complex, each new advance became more challenging. Thus, new discoveries accounted for the initial rapid growth of innovations, but the continued growth of knowledge was unable to maintain the same rate of innovation. Ongoing innovation has allowed the industry to remain strong through the development of a continuous supply of upgrades, but not to grow at its initial rate. Thus, it is not true that the growth of knowledge hindered R&D output in the microprocessor industry per se, but rather that the kind of knowledge being generated was not capable of supporting innovation at a constant rate. In other words, the relationship between knowledge growth and the rate of innovation is nonlinear and, on reflection, it would be surprising if it were. What this means is that R&D investment in one area might produce knowledge that fails to drive a high rate of innovation, but new information in a different field may be quite capable of doing so. In other words, R&D investment is only unproductive because of a failure to identify the correct area to investigate in order to obtain the knowledge needed to sustain competitive innovation. Why did Kodak continue to focus on film photography when their competitors and consumers were switching to digital? Why did Bell Laboratories continue to prioritise valve technology and permit Sony to acquire a license to work with transistors? This raises the interesting, and perhaps more important, questions: what are the characteristics of knowledge that lead to innovations and what and who determines which research avenues to pursue in order to foster new innovation? One implication is that R&D productivity declines because business systems lose the ability to target R&D investment effectively as they transform from small science-based enterprises into businesses, following their initial success.

Declining R&D Productivity and the Business Cycle

Robert Evenson examined relations between R&D productivity and several industrial economic factors over time and found that increasing demand, particularly foreign demand, was most closely associated with declining R&D productivity.[23] At first this might appear counter intuitive; we might expect greater demand for the uses of innovations to be associated with strongly competitive companies and a more productive R&D output. Indeed, many economists' early attempts to model economic growth assumed that it would have a positive impact on R&D productivity.[28,29] Why then should the reverse be the case? If we take the pharmaceutical industry, the decline in R&D productivity appears to be general and industry-wide with some variations, suggesting the role of some wide-ranging factors. It is also the case that increasing demand for its innovated products has occurred during recent decades. As discussed above, much thought has been given to the possibility that technical challenges related to advances in science and technology may be the cause. However relatively little consideration has been given to the operation of the industry itself and its business cycle, and what impact these might have on R&D capacity and productivity.

The pharmaceutical industry has been through a rapid growth phase, which is now coming to an end, if it has not already ended, and the industry finds itself at what economists refer to as the mature phase of the business cycle. This is characterised by slowing growth, accumulated cash from past success, reduction in the number of companies in the field due to mergers and acquisitions, low-grade innovations and low R&D productivity. This would seem to characterise the present state of the industry very well; if true, economic business cycle theory predicts that decline will follow. But is this inevitable? Is eventual decline built into the fabric of the industry or is it a consequence of external factors related to knowledge, science and technology?

There are many reasons why medical science and the biomedical industry should be capable of continuing to grow rather than falling victim to theoretical economic predictions of inevitable decline. It has an assured market for new and better treatments and diagnostic methods, which is certain to grow as emerging economies expand. The pharmaceutical and medical devices industries, despite frequent criticism, have proven themselves in the past to be extremely good at producing highly effective health products and there is no reason to doubt their continued capacity to do so, given the right circumstances and knowledge. The industry still has the financial strength to invest in an effective recovery. But for this to occur the industry will need to change; but where and in what direction should this change occur? The key to this may well be found in its own history, for there were fewer more successful industries in the 20th century. Reinventing the scientific culture which drove that success would seem a reasonable place to start.

Summary and Conclusions

Innovation, meaning changes to existing products or new ones that capture markets and boost sales and profits, is widely considered to be the key to economic growth and prosperity. This singular view masks the fact that some innovations, such as tobacco consumption and excessive use of fossils fuels, may be harmful to health and society in general. It also hinders a careful analysis of other contributing factors on which successful innovation depends, such as scientific discovery.

A public perception that some innovations are marketed primarily for the benefit of producers has led to mistrust in some industries, notably the nuclear power generation, genetically modified food and pharmaceutical industries. In the case of drug development and biomedical science, this has contributed to increased regulation and the greatly increased cost of developing new treatments, to a point that is not sustainable.

The pharmaceutical industry also faces a crisis due to a dramatic reduction in research productivity. This is partly explained by the huge increase in development costs, but it also reflects the prevailing narrow view of innovations as a business venture and failure to grasp the critical role that fundamental and original science plays in generating the knowledge needed to foster them. Reversing the fortunes of big pharma will require restoring biomedical science to the centre of its survival strategy; this might be achieved most easily by reinventing the scientific culture on which the pharmaceutical industry built its outstanding success during the last century.

References

1. Andersen, B., Britain must think bigger. *The Guardian*, 8 September 2011. http://www.guardian.co.uk/commentisfree/2011/sep/08/big-innovation-centre-launch. Accessed 5 July 2012.
2. Shakespeare, *Henry IV, Part 1*, Act V, Scene 1, 78.
3. Schumpeter, J.A., *Business Cycles*. McGraw-Hill, New York, 1939.
4. Allen, J.A., *Scientific Innovation and Industrial Prosperity*. Elsevier, Amsterdam, 1967.
5. Hutton, W., We are on the verge of a new age of invention. *The Times*, 8 September 2011.
6. Rogers, E.M., *Diffusion of Innovation*. Free Press, New York, 1962.
7. Lopez, A.D., Mathers, C.D., Ezzati, M., *et al.* (Eds), *Global Burden of Disease and Risk Factors*. Oxford University Press and the World Bank, Oxford, 2006.
8. Murray, C.J. and Lopez, A.D., Global mortality, disability, and the contribution of risk factors: global Burden of Disease study. *The Lancet*, 1997; 349, 1436–1442.
9. Sheron, N., Hawkey, C. and Gilmore, I., Projections of alcohol deaths: a wake-up call. *The Lancet*, 2011; 377, 1297–1299.
10. Balakrishnan, R., Allender, S., Scarborough, P., *et al.*, The burden of alcohol-related ill health in the United Kingdom. *J. Public Health*, 2009; 31(3), 366–373.
11. BMA Board of Science, Alcohol misuse: tackling the UK epidemic. February 2008. http://www.drugslibrary.stir.ac.uk/documents/alcoholmisuse.pdf. Accessed 5 July 2012.

12. Gabbey. J. and Walley, T., Introducing new health interventions. *BMJ,* 2006; 332, 64–65.

13. Rawlins, M.D., Cutting the cost of drug development? *Nature Rev. Drug Discovery,* 2004; 3, 360–363.

14. House of Lords Science and Technology Committee, Third report. February 2000. http://www.publications.parliament.uk/pa/ld199900/ldselect/ldsctech /38/3816.htm. Accessed 5 July 2012.

15. Connelly, D., Restoring public trust in pharma. PharmExec.com, 1 April 2011. http://pharmexec.findpharma.com/pharmexec/Commentary/Restoring-Public-Trust-in-Pharma/ArticleStandard/Article/detail/716295. Accessed 5 July 2012.

16. Cockburn, I.M., Is the pharmaceutical industry in a productivity crisis? in *Innovation Policy and the Economy,* Number 7. National Bureau of Economic Research and MIT Press, Cambridge, Mass., 2006. http://www.hbs.edu/ units/tom/seminars/2007/docs/Cockburn%20-%20Is%20Pharma%20in%20 a%20Productivity%20Crisis%20-%20scanned.pdf. Accessed 5 July 2012.

17. McKinnon, R., Worzel, K., Rotz, G., *et al.*, Crisis? What crisis? A fresh diagnosis of big pharma's R&D productivity crunch. Research paper from Marakon Associates, New York, 2004. http://www.marakon.com/ideas_pdf/ id_041104_mckinnon.pdf. Accessed 21 October 2008.

18. Department of Health, A new value-based approach to the pricing of branded medicines. December 2010. http://www.dh.gov.uk/prod_consum_dh/groups/ dh_digitalassets/@dh/@en/documents/digitalasset/dh_122793.pdf. Accessed 5 July 2012.

19. Mintz, C.S., Financial crisis reshaping the life sciences industry. *Science Careers,* 10 April 2009. http://sciencecareers.sciencemag.org/career_magazine/ previous_issues/articles/2009_04_10/caredit.a0900048. Accessed 5 July 2012.

20. Cures for an industry crisis: big pharma scrambles to find new ways to develop drugs faster. Knowledge @ Wharton, 10 February 2011. http://knowledge. wharton.upenn.edu/article.cfm?articleid=2709. Accessed 5 July 2012.

21. Pammolli, F., Magazzini, L. and Riccaboni, M., The productivity crisis in pharmaceutical R&D. *Nat. Rev. Drug Discov.,* 2011; 10, 428–438.

22. Helpman, E. and Trajtenberg, M., Diffusion of general purpose technologies. National Bureau of Economic Research Working Paper, 1996. http://www. nber.org/papers/w5773.pdf?new_window=1. Accessed 5 July 2012.

23. Everson, R., Patents, R&D and invention potential: international evidence. *Amer. Econ. Rev.* 1993; 83, 463–468.

24. Segerstrom, P., Endogenous growth without scale effects. *Amer. Econ. Rev.*, 1998; 88, 1290–1310.

25. Shah, A.M. and Mann, D.L., In search of new therapeutic targets and strategies for heart failure: recent advances in basic science. *The Lancet*, 2011; 378, 704–712.

26. Orsenigo, L., Pammolli, F. and Riccaboni, M., Technological change and network dynamics: lessons from the pharmaceutical industry. *Research Policy*, 2001; 30, 485–508.

27. Jones, B., The burden of knowledge and the 'death of renaissance man': is innovation getting harder? *Rev. Econ. Stud.*, 2009; 76, 283–317.

28. Romer, P.M., Endogenous technological change. *Journal of Political Economy.* 1990; 9S, S71–SI02.

29. Segerstrom P.S., Anant, T.C.A. and Dinopoulos, E., A Schumpeterian model of the product life cycle. *Amer. Econ. Rev.*, 1990; 50, 1077–1092.

9

The Centrality of Medical Science in the 21st Century: Protecting Health and Meeting Future Economic Challenges

Introduction

If a person born in the early 19th century were to return today they would be astonished by the advances in medical science that we now take for granted. Concerns about how long we may have to wait for our scan or treatment may overshadow our recognition of the outstanding achievements represented by the technology and skills involved in such procedures, but on reflection, there can be no doubt that exceptional progress has been made, particularly during the 20th century. But, as we have also seen, medical progress has begun to stall. Medical research is in decline, drug development is in crisis and there is a worrying level of public mistrust of some medical advances and of the pharmaceutical industry in particular. There is clear evidence that further great progress is possible, but paradoxically the more successful we have been the harder it seems to be to continue in that vein. Is this inevitable? Does medical progress have to follow a trajectory of development, maturity and decline as economic theory predicts for business cycles? Can the present decline in medical science be reversed, and if it can, what would it take to achieve it?

The Economics Case for Medical Research

The idea that medical science to date has achieved an acceptable level of progress and that further developments are simply adding an unacceptable increase in cost to hard-pressed health budgets is a serious question in today's economic climate. I believe the reverse is the case and that continued economic growth will increasingly depend on finding new ways to prevent and treat illness and to prolong the period of good health in peoples' lives. This is true for economies at all stages of development, but particularly so for mature economies faced with stagnant growth.

Health and Economic Growth

Economic theory suggests that businesses, industries and national economies behave according to predictable patterns. In 1959, Walt Rostow formulated economic development in a series of designated stages from the traditional society through increasing growth to a mature state characterised by high mass consumption and reduced productivity.[1] Over the past three decades, research has focused on understanding the factors which govern economic growth during the later mature phases, characterised by stable production but low growth, in order to find ways to rejuvenate that growth. Of the many factors that determine economic productivity, the characteristics of the workforce, often referred to as human capital, has received the most attention.[2] Life expectancy has long been known to be closely correlated with GDP, both because the quality of health services depend on prosperity and also because health and longevity are elements of human capital on which productivity depends; life expectancy of nations is positively related to their economic development just as, for example, the high prevalence of infectious diseases adversely impacts on it.[3] It is not difficult to envisage that economic growth is held back in countries afflicted by low survival rates and high levels of infectious diseases, such as malaria and HIV/AIDs, and that improving health and longevity in those countries would be economically advantageous.

The Malthusian Trap

In developed countries, life expectancy has increased dramatically over the past century (as discussed in Chapter 7) and this has contributed significantly to the growth they have enjoyed. Indeed some argue that population growth accounted for most of the marked increase in GDP in

England between 1700 and 1860.[4] But there is also the potential risk that rapid population growth might surpass increasing wealth and output resulting in failure to improve living standards, known as the 'Malthusian trap' after Thomas Malthus (1766–1834). Some early studies provided support for the Malthusian trap based on evidence from a wide range of countries showing GDP to be positively related to longevity up to about 60 years,[5] but reaching a plateau thereafter. This explains in part the concern in many Western countries about the rising cost of caring for their elderly populations that has led to proposals in several nations to increase the retirement age. It may also explain some negative economic views about the benefits of medical science; should we really be investing in research that will increase life expectancy further at a time when we are struggling to cope with the social and economic consequences of what has already been achieved?

In fact studies have demonstrated that the increased life expectancy observed in recent decades has not led to a Malthusian trap. Indeed the reverse has occurred; between 1966 and 1999, the world's population doubled from 3 to 6 billion but per capita income tripled.[6] Several reasons have been put forward to explain this: (i) increased longevity can lead to a longer working life, particularly if the extra years are healthy ones, (ii) increased life expectancy has been associated with higher savings rates during working life, supporting continued consumption in later life, (iii) fertility rates have declined as survival has increased resulting in greater female participation in the workforce, (iv) declining fertility rates have also been associated with greater educational attainments as parents have opted for fewer but more highly-educated children and (v) labour shortages in high-income countries have begun to oblige employers to adopt more accommodating approaches towards older workers, such as flexible working, shifting heavy physical work to younger employees and running in-house clinics and wellness programmes.[6] Thus, the contribution that medical science has made to healthier and longer lives has been associated with a substantial increase in per capita productivity. It follows that the challenge of providing care for older populations is not an issue of resource availability but one of resource distribution and that the notion of older age groups as an economic burden produced by advances in medical science is both as untrue as it is objectionable.

Cognitive Skills and Health are Essential for Economic Growth

Understanding the reasons for this unanticipated increase in productivity is important because it suggests that mature economies may be capable of breaking out of the growth stagnation predicted by economic theory. There is no doubt that improving health and longevity in low-income counties is important for their economic growth. In high-income countries, where dramatic increases in survival have already been achieved, the quality of health will be increasingly important. Studies in recent decades investigating the characteristics of human capital that determine economic productivity have identified education[3] in mathematics and languages as particularly important.[7-9] For mature economies, increasing productivity depends on finding new and more efficient ways of producing goods, for which high cognitive skill levels are important. Good health and the absence of disability are crucial in allowing people to learn and develop the skills they need and to use these skills to engage in productive work. Increased participation in the workforce in later life is already planned and will require that the extra years of life we now enjoy are also healthy and free of disability. In fact, epidemiologists have long realised that within any country the number of years lived without disability is a critical measure of public health.

When viewed in this way it is clear that the challenges facing medicine and medical research are immense and this applies equally to low- and high-income countries. Despite the marked improvements in health and longevity that have been achieved globally, huge effort is still needed in low- and middle-income countries. However, in the richest countries wide and dramatic variations in health and survival continue to exist; for example, life expectancy in the most deprived and most affluent areas in England and Wales in 1998 was 72 and 77 years respectively for men and 78 and 81 for women.[10] Reducing disability and improving the quality of health for all to enable older people to continue working beyond the traditional retirement age will be important to avoid falling living standards in the future. In economic terms, investing in medical research, particularly in relation to chronic debilitating diseases, and understanding how to improve health in later life will be important for our economic prosperity.

Challenges Facing Medical Science

To take just a few examples, mental illness inflicts decades of misery on millions of people in all regions of the world and although treatments have improved greatly in recent decades, many of them are relatively crude and often associated with undesirable side effects. Cancer will affect more people globally as longevity increases and thus remains a great challenge. Some cancers can now be cured and in certain others, such as some cases of prostate cancer, progression can be slow so that they have little impact on either survival or quality of life. Even if a cure for cancer is not possible, the ability to replicate this slow progression would have huge benefits. Hypertension is the world's greatest cause of disability.[11] In the developing world most cases go untreated, but even in the developed world treatment requires medication for life and in the majority of cases involves a combination of drugs. The benefits on a global scale of a long-term cure or prevention would be immense. In the US, 46.1 million people suffered from arthritis and other rheumatic conditions in 2003, incurring medical expenditure of $321.8 billion and earnings losses of $47 billion.[12] The economic burden of these ailments, which mainly afflict the adult working population, is set to increase as populations age. Increasing the retirement age of the workforce can only be effective if good health is maintained in later life and this means finding new ways to prevent and treat many of our common chronic diseases. I have no doubt that many of these conditions will one day be largely preventable through better understanding of their causes and the discovery of new treatments. This progress will only come about through investment in research.

This might seem obvious, but already there are signs that a contrary view operates in some areas of public health policy. Thus, in contrast to the global approach to HIV/AIDs, where a broad strategy which includes intensive medical research is strongly encouraged and supported, public health ambitions for dealing with the far greater and neglected challenges of non-communicable diseases focus on social interventions such as modification of diet, weight reduction and exercise, to the virtual exclusion of medical research and medical treatment.[13] The recent WHO report, World Health Statistics 2011, failed to even mention medical conditions such as hypertension,[14] currently the most important cause of disability in the world.[15] Clearly social conditions have an important impact on health, but for global organisations like the UN and WHO to ignore the role that medicine and medical science can play in tackling global health problems is damaging, not only to our ability to deal with such problems effectively, but also to our ability to conduct medical research and risks inflicting lasting damage. For the reasons discussed above, it also has serious consequences for our long-term economic development.

The Malthusian trap has been avoided in the developed Western world so far by increasing the productivity of human capital, mainly by harnessing cognitive skills through enlightened policies of education.[9] As the impact of aging demographics increases, some large countries with ample space may continue to rely on a steady flow of educated immigrants, as the US has done so successfully. However this is a limited option in many European countries where the challenge will be to make better use of the existing workforce by prolonging working lives and enhancing the value of work done. This can only be achieved by improving the health of older people, reducing the years lived with disability and understanding in much greater detail the effects of working on physical and mental health.

There are now indications that the need to improve the health of older people is being recognised.[16] Thus, the economic case for medical research is clear and the potential benefits immense. Improving health will be fundamental for future economic prosperity. This means reversing the woeful state of health in low-income countries and getting to grips with the long-neglected burden of chronic disease in both low- and high-income countries. It also means improving the health of older populations, for which new and better long-term preventive and curative treatments will be needed.

Research Productivity

A recent analysis from the US National Science Foundation showed that the number of papers published in the fields of science and engineering changed little between 1990 and 2003, yet R&D funding increased by around 60%. A notable factor within the data was a negative association between the number of scientists with medical degrees and output; publication counts increased for post-doctorate scientists without medical degrees in contrast to a decrease for medics.[17] Scientific research is a major contributor to economic prosperity and achieving a good return on investment in science is important. Just as health and education are recognised as important for economic development, understanding the factors which determine research productivity is also important for our future prosperity. What makes a good scientist? What motivates people? Can science be organised and managed so as to improve productivity? This last question is particularly important for medical science, where the decline in productivity has been steeper than in other areas.

The level of cognitive skills in a population is recognised as important for economic development. This is true in relation to the average attainment achieved in science, maths and language, but recent evidence also suggests that the percentage of a population reaching the highest levels of attainment is an even greater determinant of GDP.[9] There is clearly something special about the skills and drive that has allowed our greatest scientists to make the groundbreaking discoveries for which they are renowned. What are they and what are the conditions in which they flourish? High levels of achievement in the traditional measures of educational attainment would be expected, but something beyond this must surely be needed.

There are many scientists one could call on to illustrate the qualities of such men and women. The year 2015 will mark the second centenary of the achievement of one of our less-remembered but nevertheless most remarkable scientists. In 1815, William Smith published his geological map of England and in doing so created the new science of geology, forever changing our understanding of how the Earth was formed. Geology challenged the traditional (and strongly held) biblical view of the Earth as powerfully as did Charles Darwin's *On the Origin of Species*, and it did so 44 years before that famous publication. Darwin's impact was greater because it caused outrage at the time by suggesting that humans evolved from animals, but Smith's discoveries about the origins of the Earth were arguably of equal importance.

What Makes a Great Scientist?

Characteristics of Great Scientists

• Highly curious
• Clever, observant
• Capable of holding and integrating large amounts of information
• Single-minded
• Independently-minded
• Determined and tenacious
• Motivated by
   o Curiosity
   o Abstract rewards (the esteem of peers)

William Smith's life, described by Simon Winchester in *The Map that Changed the World*,[18] seems to me to be of particular interest because it illustrates some of the key attributes of a great scientist. He was born in 1769 in Oxfordshire, the son of a blacksmith. After the death of his father when he was 8 years old, Smith went to live with his uncle, who farmed locally. Smith appears to have been an observant boy and developed an interest in the local habit of collecting poundstones (so named because their regular size, shape and mass made them useful as simple weights in farm dairies), also known as Chedworth buns. They were in fact fossils of the echinoid *Clypeus ploti* and were a common finding in the fields around his uncle's farm. Smith's formal education was modest and did not include university, but he kept diaries which reveal an exceptional and growing interest in what lay beneath the ground. For most of his life he collected and named hundreds of fossils and he realised that the Earth's strata could be identified from the fossils found in them.

Working as a canal builder and on land drainage, he noticed regular patterns to the strata across the country and around 1798 he conceived the idea of making a great map of the stratigraphy of the entire country. He became passionate, some would say obsessed, about this aim and spent almost 20 years collecting the information that would be the basis of his map as he travelled around the country doing his paid work. Smith finally published his map in 1815, having undertaken this work at his own expense and to the neglect of his own security. He fell into debt and was imprisoned for it in the King's Bench Prison in London in 1819. The Geological Society initially refused to acknowledge his work and it was not until 1831 that, with the support of more enlightened scientists, the Geological Society publicly acknowledged his work by awarding him its first Wollaston Medal; the following year he received a pension from the government.

Smith's contribution was of the highest rank; working alone he laid the foundation for a new science. His achievement helpfully illustrates some of the attributes of great scientists. He was not educated formally to a high level, but he was clever and highly observant. He had a mind capable of holding large quantities of information and examining that information in a rational way that allowed him to see a structure of the Earth that the generations before him had failed to notice. He was utterly persistent and determined, driven by a combination of curiosity and a deep attraction to the beauty of the picture which was unfolding in his mind. He was single-minded and independently-minded in pursuing the trail that would provide the information he needed. He was also highly ambitious; he badly wanted to be acknowledged by society for his work and was crushed by the initial reaction of the Geological Society. This desire to be acknowledged for his work appears to have been at least as important as profit or wealth in motivating him. Smith's social origins, his lack of formal education or a personal fortune, and his inability to write well contributed to the difficulties he experienced in publishing his work. But importantly they did not prevent him from completing the task he set himself; rather, they underline the strength of the qualities that drove him. I suggest that these are characteristics found in most great scientists and to varying degrees in many scientists committed to original scientific enquiry. As academia and industry struggle with declining research productivity it seems appropriate to consider how such individuals would fare in the world of science today.

Scientists in the 21ˢᵗ Century

The pharmaceutical industry achieved great success in the 20th century, both in the range of drugs developed and also in becoming one of our wealthiest industries, but it now struggles, with a marked decline in research productivity. Could it be that the very success the industry achieved contributed to a changed environment that makes scientific discovery more difficult? There are several reasons why this may be the case.

Managed Efficiency Versus Curiosity

As discussed in Chapter 5, drug development costs have ballooned dramatically in recent years to around $1 billion today. Companies are under enormous pressure to achieve regulatory approval as quickly as possible in order to recoup their costs before patents expire. In such an environment it is easy to understand that the focus of research will be on providing data to support safety and efficacy and that efficient management of this will be of the greatest importance for the success of the business. It is also easy to understand that an individual captivated and driven by an intense curiosity about a scientific question that is not aligned with the company's business plans would struggle in such an environment.

Secrecy Versus Open Discourse

Success in the industry depends on protection of information property, which in some companies may reflect more than half the capital value of the company. This can draw a cloud of secrecy over research undertaken and restrict its publication so as to protect patent rights. The normal discourse that surrounds scientific investigation is therefore controlled and limited, which not only hinders potential competitors, but also the researchers involved.

Financial Reward Versus Public Approbation

Secrecy also means that scientists have little chance of public approbation. Of course, industry can and does reward success financially, but this misses what may in fact be of even greater importance for many scientists. For example, Darwin wrote, 'my love of natural science has been ... much aided by the ambition to be esteemed by my fellow naturalists.'[19] William Smith drove himself and his family into debt and prison in order to achieve his research objective. Such behaviour might initially appear out of place in today's economic climate, but it should not. After all, many scientists spend much their lives captivated by ideas and concepts and it should therefore not be surprising that the rewards they most covet are equally abstract.

Team Working Versus Individualism

It is a common feature of the business environment that successful workers are promoted to increasingly managerial roles. As a consequence, the industry may appear less attractive to individuals with scientific talent. Successful scientists tend to be single-minded and determined, whereas the efficiency which industry seeks to achieve is more often structured around teams working along agreed pathways backed by regular performance measurements.

Thus, one of the reasons big pharma has become less successful in making new discoveries is because it has created a culture which is less conducive to original science. This has partly arisen due to its own past history but also because of efforts to overcome the rising costs of drug development. The huge investments it has made in high tech facilities, ring-fenced behind walls of secrecy, are simply less conducive to scientific discovery than the traditional open ways of science. Too many of the scientists who enter the industry emerge as managers or public relations officers. Changing the culture that has created this scenario will be immensely challenging for the industry, and perhaps impossible. It is clear however that the present system has not worked. Companies are having to downsize[20,21] as the scientific breakthroughs on which they depend have failed to materialise. But reducing costs will only work in the short term and further contraction is inevitable unless more effective ways of doing research can be found. Some have recommended closer collaboration with smaller and more innovative companies, particularly in the development of new gene-based products. But this too has largely disappointed, partly because the need to make a rapid breakthrough before the start-up investment capital is exhausted obliges such small companies to pursue even more aggressively-managed research programmes aimed at rapid regulatory approval, which leaves little room for any curiosity-driven science.

Signs of Change?

This situation will have to change if the industry is going to be able to rejuvenate its ability to develop new therapeutic pathways. A new culture that encourages and harnesses those human talents and attributes that motivate good science will have to be created. Some recent developments suggest that a growing realisation of the necessity for change may be dawning on the industry as companies seek to ditch the old in-house directed research approach in favour of a more outward-looking and open strategy. This may be behind moves to form closer collaborations with academia. Some of the largest players, such as Pfizer, GlaxoSmithKline and AstraZeneca, have recently established agreements with several large academic institutions which are reminiscent of those that existed during the 1960s and 1970s, in which they provide research funding and an unprecedented sharing of scientific information[22] in the hope of rejuvenating discovery, while closing large segments of their in-house research laboratories. This is undoubtedly a hopeful sign for the industry, although painful for the staff involved in the in-house closures. There will be many fingers crossed in the boardrooms of pharmaceutical companies as executives hope that academia can deliver the new avenues for drug development they need. Academia has been successful in providing the knowledge base for discoveries in the past; can academia do it again now?

Can Academia Deliver?

Research carried out in academic institutions has traditionally been based on open peer reviewed publication and it will be important for this process to be maintained in the new collaborative centres supported by industry. Initial reports suggest that broad publication rights will be maintained and that the new collaborations will share information property. There are some potential concerns however. Universities have also been exposed to increasing economic pressures in recent years and have reacted by adopting some of the behaviours of industry. For example, in recent years universities have sought to optimise the value of information property as the pharmaceutical industry has done. This approach has seen a dramatic increase in patents awarded to US medical schools between 1976 and 2003,[23] and Europe, Japan and China are following the same path. This is entirely understandable from an economic perspective, but it also means a general increase in closed research or a delay in publication needed to protect property rights, which runs counter to the needs of science. Furthermore, research productivity has also been declining in academia and this has been more marked for medical research than other areas of science.[17] The challenges facing academic medicine are formidable, as discussed in Chapter 1. The sharp decline in numbers of clinical academics and the increasing difficulty in conducting research in clinical settings embroiled in cycles of economic and managerial reforms have pushed medical science to the margins. And of course academic institutions have been obliged to invest in administrative resources to manage the citation metrics to which their funding is tied. Medical journals that were once devoted to publishing articles on medical science are transformed into magazines containing opinions, news, letters, clinical guidelines, audits, re-analysis of earlier studies, performance measurements and obituaries.[24]

There is an urgent need to reinvigorate and support medical science starting at the bedside and in the clinic. This in turn will require that the real value of such science is understood. As discussed in Chapter 5, the narrow accountancy approach of citation measurements fails to capture the value of clinical science and has contributed to its marginalisation by academic institutions focused on league tables of performance. This needs to be abandoned or developed into a system that captures research value in a more meaningful way. Figure 9.1 shows a model of medical science to illustrate its wide range of interactions, the support that drives it and its contributions to knowledge and health. Viewed in this way, the limitations of the citation approach to measuring value in medical science become clear. Publications are undoubtedly an important aspect of its output, but just one of many. Medical science's role in educating future scientists and contributing to the knowledge base are also important. An active research capacity in the context of clinical practice is also essential to help direct basic science into relevant areas and to identify opportunities and new challenges as well as to evaluate the safety and efficacy of new treatments. Medical science has also made important rediscoveries of old remedies. For example, the discovery of the mode of action of aspirin in 1972 and the importance of thrombosis in vascular diseases led to the drug's rediscovery as an important treatment to prevent heart attacks. Similarly, an active science base in medicine was important in identifying new clinical applications for discoveries, such as ultrasound and X-rays, in other sciences. Medical science has also played a vital and leading role in the discovery of many clinical inventions, such as artificial joints. The current

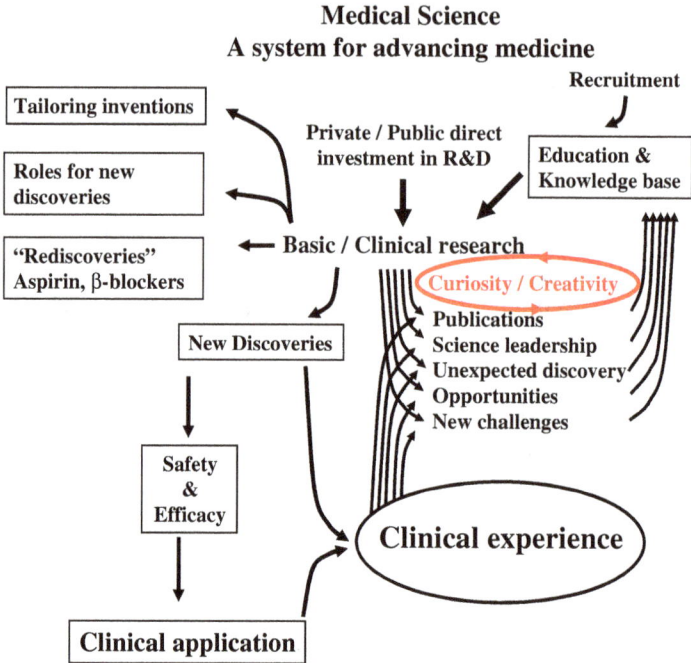

Figure 9.1. The process of discovery in medical science requires a two way interaction between clinical and basic research which harnesses the curiosity and creativity arising from clinical practice. Its outputs include growing the knowledge base and educating young clinical scientists to maintain the science capacity for the future, finding new uses for previous discoveries based on new knowledge, capturing unexpected discoveries and identifying discoveries in other areas of science to meet clinical needs. Viewed in this way it is clear that the capacity to do medical science has immense value that goes far beyond what can be measured by citation metrics.

approach of science measurement all too often captures the new product or invention but forgets the value of the processes which created it.

The current anxiety about bacterial resistance to antibiotics illustrates the weakness of this approach. We are rightly concerned about overuse of antibiotics, but it is only a matter of time before bacteria develop resistance to most antibiotics and the only way forward is to continue to study the process by which they do so and to develop new ways to target them. We have to regard science as an ongoing and central asset for protecting health and meeting the inevitable health challenges that will arise in the future, not something that can be dispensed with once it has delivered some new wonder drug.

Sunset?

Whatever the economic pressures facing health care delivery, abandoning original clinical research will be far more costly in the long term. A thriving clinical science base is essential to generating a culture of enquiry related to medicine and to keeping biomedical science grounded and relevant to understanding disease, its diagnosis and treatment. Without this, biological science may still flourish, citation indices may still perform well, but it will continue to struggle to be clinically relevant; citations don't cure or feed people. This will be the toughest challenge facing medical science in the coming decades. The sunset scenario is one in which the leadership of medicine is drawn into the political and economic struggle about how health care is provided, the value of science is overshadowed by competition between providers based on short-term selective efficiencies and a work-force increasingly tied to delivery performance. Over time, with less clinical science being undertaken and academic posts left vacant, the culture of enquiry is diminished and new generations of clinicians are trained in an environment focused exclusively on delivery, performance and audit. The end would be that individuals gifted with the aptitudes for scientific enquiry begin to see medicine as a restrictive career and are drawn to more inquisitive and open sciences.

A New Dawn?

The extensive damage being inflicted by the present decline will have to be understood and action taken to reverse it if medical science is to be rejuvenated. This would need a new approach to measuring the wider value of medical science and abandoning the selective short-term account-ancy of citation metrics, which serves only to give administrators and managers a sense of control. The booming citation metrics in biological sciences belies the real damage being inflicted on medical science as it continues its long gradual decline. The serious difficulties facing the phar-maceutical industry and the failure of the new biologies to deliver the advances hoped for, despite huge investment, should serve as a wake-up call. New collaborations being built between academia and industry are intended to include clinical science, which may be an indication of real insight; but this will need to be solidly based in the clinic if it is to succeed. Academic institutions too need to understand and value their clinical partners. Research funds for biomedical science will not last if all there is to show for it is citation metrics. Unless the 'medical' component becomes something more tangible, sooner or later citation metrics will come to be seen as the emperor's new clothes.

The challenges facing medical science that I have outlined in this book are formidable, but there are many reasons for optimism and I am firmly of the view that they can and will be overcome. This might seem surprising to some readers, but, just as it is true that advances in medicine begin by understanding the nature of the illness, so too, in considering the future of medical science itself, it is necessary to start by examining the nature and causes of the challenges it faces. Furthermore, despite the radical upheavals of recent years, medicine also has many formidable strengths.

Our Best Students and an Adaptive Science-based Curriculum

Medicine continues to attract many of our brightest students, who continue to receive a broad education that includes a strong element of science. The curriculum has adapted in positive ways to meet advances in medicine and the changing medical needs of patients. In addition, the selection of students has adapted rapidly to reflect current social conditions, such as achieving gender equality. The potential of our young clinicians to respond to the medical challenges is as great today as it has ever been.

Strong Ethical Foundations

Medicine continues to be based on a strong ethical foundation. Challenges to medical professionalism in recent decades have been met with a renewed global commitment.[25] Medicine globally has maintained a strong stand against, and has been critical of, individual doctors who have participated in torture or in carrying out death sentences. As I write, the new emerging ethical challenge is likely to be the question of assisted suicide and whether doctors should help people in the act of ending their own lives. Balancing the need to protect the vulnerable from direct or indirect coercion and providing adequate relief from suffering for patients who are ill with due attention to the risks and benefits of analgesia are extremely complex questions, and are far removed from the narrow framework of personal choice in which medical ethics is often shrouded. The profession wisely maintains a steady course in deliberating on such matters, reflecting on and learning from its long experience over many generations in meeting the immediate needs of today. This is also important for medical science since it needs to be based within clinical practice and therefore needs the trust and confidence of the public. The available evidence indicates that clinicians do continue to be held in high regard.

The Clinician–Patient Relationship

Caring for patients involves a highly complex set of experiences. Clinicians are constantly aware of the physical and psychological suffering of their patients. Each new diagnosis brings to mind the strengths and limitations of their personal knowledge as well as those of current medical practice. Medicine has achieved many spectacular cures, but many treatments also carry risks of serious side effects or may have to be taken for life. Thus, medical practice, through the empathy it engenders and its inherent limitations, is itself a powerful driver to think about and search for better ways to care for people. It is for this reason that the clinician–patient relationship, in the context of high standards of medical professionalism, has been important in driving medical research in the past. By its nature, medical practice will always require a high level of personal contact and this will ensure that it continues to be a powerful impetus for medical research in the future.

Reform and Adapt Transparently

In recent decades, examples of medical misdeeds and the serious criminal activity of a few individuals have led to harsh criticisms of the way doctors are regulated and to calls for reform. On the whole, regulatory bodies have responded positively and transparently to these and this ability to adapt and reform has undoubtedly contributed to the high level of public confidence medicine continues to have.

Much of the upheaval in health care over the past two decades, which has disrupted clinical science, has been driven ultimately by contrary economic views; on the one hand, medical science is seen as something that adversely drives up health care costs, while on the other, it is regarded as a vital component of one of our most important industries. In recent years, the former view has been dominant, but as is now acknowledged that this has been at serious cost to the latter. Resolving this contradiction will be important in restoring medical science to its former position at the heart of the life sciences. Economic reflexes are slow to operate. Nevertheless, recent years have witnessed remarkable changes in our willingness to invest in reversing global health inequalities and, apart from the moral reasons for this, there are also clear-headed political and economic arguments. In the same way, finding new and better ways to improve life-long disability-free health in high-income countries will come to be seen as an essential element in strategies for promoting economic growth. Medical science has proved its ability to deliver advances that have transformed health in just a couple of generations in ways our grandparents would have had difficulty imagining possible. It has the ability to continue to do this so long as there are people willing and able to ask how and why.

Summary and Conclusions

The increased financial and economic pressures on health care delivery have been major contributors to the marginalisation and decline of medical science over the past three decades as health systems have undergone reforms aimed at containing and reducing costs. However, economic growth in the longer term will increasingly depend on finding ways to increase per capita productivity and this will require increasing the average level of cognitive skills and improving the health of the workforce. Increasing the working life of people requires not only that we live longer, but also that we are healthy and free of disability during those extra years. This represents an immense challenge to medical science. The global burden of chronic diseases is now recognised as our greatest health challenge as life expectancy has increased in most regions of the world. It is also one which has been neglected for several decades, but will need to be addressed if present ambitions to increase the working lives of people are to be realised. This will not be possible without a major reinvigoration of medical science.

The marked decline in research productivity in the pharmaceutical industry in recent decades reflects a sharp increase in the cost of meeting regulatory requirements, but the failure to fill companies' pipelines with adequate supplies of new and profitable drugs is ultimately due to a failure of scientific discovery. The latter reflects a failed model of conducting science. Efficient direction of technology, however sophisticated, to meet goals determined by market needs in a culture of secrecy is not conducive to original science. Recent moves by the industry to form collaborations with academia reminiscent of the relationship that existed in the middle of the 20th century suggest that this has now been realised, and may represent a turning point.

Whether these collaborations succeed will depend on how academia responds for it too has changed radically over the past few decades. Faced with increasing economic challenges, academia has taken on some of the behaviours of industry with a sharp increase in patent applications and information property protection in recent years, with the danger that publications and knowledge-sharing may be inhibited. For academic medicine there is the risk that ongoing tensions over health budgets may obscure the central role that medical science plays in meeting future challenges, with the result that it continues to be marginalised as an unaffordable luxury.

There are signs that these dangers are at last being recognised. Global health inequalities are now seen to be a major obstacle to economic development and political stability, and this is driving important changes. Mature economies faced with the alarming costs of caring for their aging populations have recognised that meeting this challenge requires people to have longer working lives and this will not be possible without major advances in treatment and prevention of chronic diseases. It is to be hoped that the new collaborations between industry and academia will initiate medical research that addresses real health issues arising from clinical experience and do not become just another opportunity to score citation metrics. It seems clear that the economic, social and health pressures we now face will eventually force a rejuvenation of medical science. It remains to be seen how long it will take for the pendulum to swing.

References

1. Rostow, W.W., The stages of economic growth. *Econ. Hist. Rev.*, 1959; 12(1), 1–16.
2. Romer, P., Human capital and growth: theory and evidence. *Carnegie-Rochester Conference Series on Public Policy*, 1990; 32, 2512–2586.
3. Sala-i-Martin, X., Doppelhoffer, G. and Miller, R.I., Determinants of long term growth: a Bayesian averaging of classical estimates (BACE) approach. *Amer. Econ. Rev.*, 2004; 94(4), 813–835.
4. Clark, G., *A Farewell to Alms, A Brief Economic History of the World.* Princeton University Press, Princeton, 2007.
5. Preston, S.H., The changing relation between mortality and level of economic development. *Int. J. Epidemiol.*, 2007; 36, 484–490.
6. Bloom, D.E., Canning, D. and Fink, G., Implications of population aging for economic growth. Program on the Global Demography of Aging, Working Paper 64. January 2011. http://www.hsph.harvard.edu/pgda/working.html #2011. Accessed 5 July 2012.
7. Hanushek, E.A. and Kimko, D.D., Schooling, labour-force quality and the growth of nations. *Amer. Econ. Rev.*, 2000; 90, 1184–1208.
8. Rindermann, H., Relevance of education and intelligence at the national level for the economic welfare of people. *Intelligence,* 2000; 36, 127-142.
9. Hanushek, E.A. and Woessman, L., How much do educational outcomes matter in OECD countries? *Economic Policy*, 2011; 427–491.
10. Woods, L.M., Rachet, B., Riga, M., *et al.*, Geographical variation in life expectancy at birth in England and Wales is largely explained by deprivation. *J. Epidemiol. Community Health*, 2005; 59, 115–120.
11. Lopez, A.D., Mathers, C.D., Ezzati, M., *et al.*, Global and regional burden of disease and risk factors, 2001: systematic analysis of population health data. *The Lancet,* 2006; 367, 1747–1757.
12. Yelin, E., Murphy, L., Cisternas, M.G., *et al.*, Medical care expenditures and earnings losses among persons with arthritis and other rheumatic conditions in 2003, and comparisons with 1997. *Arthritis Rheum.*, 2007; 56(5), 1397–1407.
13. United Nations preparatory papers ahead of High-level Meeting on Non-communicable Diseases held in September 2011. http://www.un.org/en/ga/president/65/issues/ncdiseases.shtml. Accessed 4 July 2012.
14. WHO, World Health Statistics. Geneva. http://www.who.int/gho/publications/world_health_statistics/en/index.html. Accessed 4 July 2012.

15. WHO, Global status report on non-communicable diseases 2010. April 2011. http://www.who.int/nmh/publications/ncd_report2010/en/. Accessed 4 July 2012.

16. Loch, C.H., Sting, F.J., Bauer, N., *et al.*, How BMW is defusing the demographic time bomb. *Harvard Business Review*, March 2010; 99–102.

17. Javitz, H., Grimes, T., Hill, D., *et al.*, U.S. academic scientific publishing. National Science Foundation Working Paper SRS 11-201, November 2010. http://www.nsf.gov/statistics/srs11201/. Accessed 4 July 2012.

18. Winchester, S., *The Map that Changed the World*. Penguin/Viking, London, 2001.

19. Barlow, N., *The Autobiography of Charles Darwin 1809–1882*. Collins, London, 1958. http://darwin-online.org.uk/majorworks.html. Accessed 4 July 2012.

20. Arnold, M., Deep cuts at AstraZeneca, Sepracor. *Medical Marketing and Media*, 29 January 2009. http://www.mmm-online.com/deep-cuts-at-astrazeneca-sepracor/article/126557/. Accessed 4 July 2012.

21. Arnold, M., Pfizer shrinks R&D operations. *Medical Marketing and Media*, 9 November 2009. http://www.mmm-online.com/pfizer-shrinks-rd-operations/article/157434/. Accessed 4 July 2012.

22. Pharmaceutical industry seeks stronger ties with academia in bid to speed up drug development. *Scientific American*, 22 June 2011. http://www.scientificamerican.com/article.cfm?id=pharmaceutical-industry-seek. Accessed 4 July 2012.

23. Azoulay, P., Michigan, R. and Sampat, B.N., The anatomy of medical school patenting. *New Eng. J. Med.*, 2007; 357, 2049–2056.

24. Godlee, F., Welcome to the new design. *BMJ*, 2011; 343, 964.

25. Medical professionalism in the new millennium: a physicians' charter. *The Lancet*, 2002; 359, 520–522.

Index

www.ingramcontent.com/pod-product-compliance
Lightning Source LLC
Chambersburg PA
CBHW050627190326
41458CB00008B/2166